The International Behavioural and Social Sciences Library

ATTENTION AND
INTERPRETATION

T0187651

TAVISTOCK

PSYCHOLOGY
In 11 Volumes

ATTENTION AND INTERPRETATION

A Scientific Approach to Insight in Psycho-Analysis and Groups

W R BION

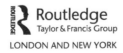

Routledge
Taylor & Francis Group

LONDON AND NEW YORK

First published in 1970 by
Tavistock Publications Limited

Reprinted in 2001 by
Routledge
2 Park Square, Milton Park, Abingdon, Oxon, OX14 4RN
711 Third Avenue, New York, NY 10017
Transferred to Digital Printing 2007

Routledge is an imprint of the Taylor & Francis Group
First issued in paperback 2013
© 1970 W R Bion

The publishers have made every effort to contact authors/copyright holders
of the works reprinted in the *International Behavioural and Social Sciences
Library*. This has not been possible in every case, however, and we would
welcome correspondence from those individuals/companies we have been
unable to trace.

These reprints are taken from original copies of each book. In many cases
the condition of these originals is not perfect. The publisher has gone to
great lengths to ensure the quality of these reprints, but wishes to point
out that certain characteristics of the original copies will, of necessity, be
apparent in reprints thereof.

British Library Cataloguing in Publication Data
A CIP catalogue record for this book
is available from the British Library

ISBN13: 978-0-415-26481-5 (hbk)

ISBN13: 978-0-415-84615-8 (pbk)

THE GRID

	Defini-tory Hypo-theses **1**	ψ **2**	Nota-tion **3**	Atten-tion **4**	Inquiry **5**	Action **6**	**. . . n**
A β-elements	A1	A2				A6	
B α-elements	B1	B2	B3	B4	B5	B6	. . . Bn
C Dream Thoughts Dreams, Myths	C1	C2	C3	C4	C5	C6	. . . Cn
D Pre-conception	D1	D2	D3	D4	D5	D6	. . . Dn
E Conception	E1	E2	E3	E4	E5	E6	. . . En
F Concept	F1	F2	F3	F4	F5	F6	. . . Fn
G Scientific Deductive System		G2					
H Algebraic Calculus							

Attention and Interpretation

A SCIENTIFIC APPROACH TO INSIGHT
IN PSYCHO-ANALYSIS AND GROUPS

W. R. BION
D.S.O., B.A., M.R.C.S., L.R.C.P.

TAVISTOCK PUBLICATIONS

LONDON · SYDNEY · TORONTO · WELLINGTON

First published in 1970
by Tavistock Publications Limited
2 Park Square, Milton Park, Abingdon, Oxon, OX14 4RN
Set in Photon Times 12 on 13 pt. by
Richard Clay (The Chaucer Press) Ltd., Bungay, Suffolk

© W. R. Bion, 1970

SBN 422 73370 9

Contents

Contents

1 · Introduction

I doubt if anyone but a practising psycho-analyst can understand this book although I have done my best to make it simple. Any psycho-analyst who is *practising* can grasp my meaning because he, unlike those who only read or hear *about* psycho-analysis, has the opportunity to experience for himself what I in this book can only represent by words and verbal formulations designed for a different task. They were developed from a background of sensuous experience. Reason is emotion's slave and exists to rationalize emotional experience. Sometimes the function of speech is to communicate experience to another; sometimes it is to miscommunicate experience to another. Sometimes the object is to achieve access to, and permit access from, a good spirit; conversely, to deny access to a bad spirit. The vocabulary forged from such material serves, though inadequately, when, as in psycho-analytic practice, the object being studied is present. In mathematics, calculations can be made without the presence of the objects about which calculation is necessary, but in psycho-analytic practice it is essential for the psycho-analyst to be able to demonstrate as he formulates. This is not possible the moment the conditions for psycho-analysis, in the narrow technical sense, do not exist. Some of us have sought to extend psycho-analytic method so that it can be employed in a group setting. Such a development, if it can be done without mutilation of the fundamental character of psycho-analytic method, would initiate the change from private to public communication. Language does just that in the domain of sensible experience. Poetic and religious expressions have made possible a degree of 'public-ation' in that formulations exist which have achieved durability and extensibility. To say the same thing differently,

1

the carrying power of the statement has been extended in time and in space. *Vixere fortes ante Agamemnona multi* and 'Not marble, nor the guilded monuments / Of princes, shall outlive this powerful rhyme' are expressions of that belief; they are interpretations of human experience. In his sphere the psycho-analyst's attention is arrested by a particular experience to which he would draw the attention of the analysand. To do this he must employ the Language of Achievement. That is to say, he must employ methods which have the counterpart of durability or extension in a domain where there is no time or space as those terms are used in the world of sense.

What I have said with regard to this book also applies to the psycho-analytic session; it is certainly my impression that the experience of psycho-analysis is supposed or intended to have an enduring effect. Unlike this book the session affords me and others an opportunity for drawing attention to the actual phenomena to which I think the analysand should attend and this might reinforce the effect of my communication. A similar advantage seems to me to be available in a psycho-analytic approach to groups; it is possible to hope that the capacity of the artist, though useful, may not be essential to the psycho-analyst. Indeed, it may be a disadvantage in so far as the artist's capacity may enable him to provide, as Plato feared, a *substitute* for the truth.

In this book I have made a few tentative approaches to a matter which I think has not received proper attention in psycho-analysis, namely, lying. The disposition to lie may be regarded as a sympton of a severely disordered personality. It certainly contributes many difficulties to any attempt at a psycho-analytic approach, but on the other hand my experience of psycho-analysis makes me feel that the aptitude for lying, so universal that only a liar could disregard its all-pervading nature, has its own place as an object for study and is ignored at a dangerous cost to analyst and analysand. In short, I agree that it is often a symptom of a disordered personality but submit that it is not necessarily a contraindication for analysis. Here I can only indicate one or two aspects.

It is too often forgotten that the gift of speech, so centrally employed, has been elaborated as much for the purpose of concealing thought by dissimulation and lying as for the purpose of elucidating or communicating thought. Therefore, the Language of Achievement, if it is to be employed for elucidating the truth, must be recognized as deriving not only from sensuous experience but also from impulses and dispositions far from those ordinarily associated with scientific discussion. Freud, like others before him, felt the need to isolate himself – insulate himself? – from the group in order to work. This would mean insulating ourselves against the very material we should study. We should, therefore, reorientate our views on such matters as rationalization and the employment of reason generally. The patient says, 'Suddenly, just as I finished lunch he threw a mug of beer in my face without any warning. I kept my head and showed no resentment at all remembering what you had said about psycho-analysis. So it passed off without anyone noticing.' Is he lying? Is he verbalizing a present hallucination? Matters of this kind are occurring throughout a psycho-analysis and demand correct assessment by the psycho-analyst. Yet we have not elaborated instruments – I have tried to do so with the grid [1] – for making the assessment. I am not speaking of making the *interpretation* or of the many theories that facilitate the making of an interpretation; the grid is of a different category altogether, analogous to a ruler in physical science, formed from a matrix of theories to aid observation and not as a substitute for observation. I commend to others a proper study of the lie and its differential diagnosis from phenomena which appear similar. The psycho-analyst must employ the Language of Achievement, but he must remember that the language was elaborated as much for the achievement of deception and evasion as for truth. This

[1] See frontispiece, and *Elements of psycho-analysis* (Bion, 1963), where the grid system is more fully discussed.

aspect is particularly clear when the prevalent emotional field is one of rivalry and hostility such as I have described, in group situations, as peculiar to the fight–flight basic assumption (Bion, 1961). The individual is similarly affected by the *group* emotional situation. It is, therefore, impossible to give correct interpretations, save by accident, unless that *situation* is assessed. For example, drug addiction is exploited as a cover for psychosis, lying is often excused as an aspect of drug addiction, and vice versa.

Psycho-analysts should determine whether they are talking of means of communication, including verbal communications, as things-in-themselves or whether they are talking of other things-in-themselves which these communication elements, gestures, actions, silences, and verbal formulations, are being used to represent. The grid is intended to remind the psycho-analyst that it is necessary to discriminate one element in his psycho-analytic experience from another and, in particular, to recognize that what matters is both the communication and the use to which it is being put. He must observe whether the presenting feature (or the feature to the obtrusion of which he wants to draw attention) is intended to further illumination or deception, and where in the genetic spectrum it belongs (primitive communication or sophisticated).

Although the grid is unsatisfactory in its present form, it will not, I hope, mislead but lead to an improved version. I have used the following signs:[1]

T — transformation
Tα — the point from which the transformation starts
Tβ — the point at which the transformation is presumed to be complete
Ta — the psycho-analyst's transformation
Tp — the analysand's transformation
O — the experience (thing-in-itself)

Analogies are frequently used. The things used and what those things represent are dissimilar. It is supposed that a

[1] Originally in *Transformations* (Bion, 1965).

4

rifle and a penis are similar. But what should be exact is the *relationship* between the particular objects in the particular analogy and not the objects themselves. Thus: as the breast is to the baby's mouth so the surgeon's knife is to the X. In any particular instance the inexactitude of the *relationship* merits criticism and appraisal. The objects are faulty and to be condemned if they *are* similar. For example, 'The knife is to the fork as the knife is to the fork' is a 'non-analogy'. 'The eyes are to the mind as the mouth is to the food' is a correct analogy and draws attention to the matter that is to be observed, namely, the relationship between the two.

2 · Medicine as a Model

Most people think of psycho-analysis, as Freud did, as a method of treatment for a complaint. The complaint was regarded as similar to a physical ailment which, when you know what it is, has to be treated in accordance with the rules of medicine. The parallel with medicine was, and still is, useful. But as psycho-analysis has grown so it has been seen to differ from physical medicine until the gap between them has passed from the obvious to the unbridgeable. For most purposes the similarity yields illuminating comparisons and models that facilitate discussion. But the more we see of psycho-analysis the more the models become inadequate to define, report, or apply psycho-analysis. Differentiation has meant that models which were illuminating have become opaque and often misleading even to psychoanalysts. Let us see why. We may start by discussing the obvious and simple reasons, though they will not remain either for long.

In physical medicine the patient may have a pain in his chest for which he can go to his doctor. To him he can explain its nature and its history and from him he can receive instructions to undergo further examination, say, by X-rays or microscopy, or certain forms of treatment. Or so it appears; later we may have reason to question this account. For the present it will serve to point the divergence of physical medicine and psycho-analysis.

Suppose the patient complained not of physical but of mental pain; no one doubts the existence of anxiety or sees any incongruity in seeking help to cure it. We find it necessary to differentiate between the pain of a broken leg and the pain, say, of bereavement; sometimes we prefer not to, but exchange mental for physical pain and vice versa. Physician

6

and psycho-analyst are alike in considering that the disease should be recognized by the physician; in psycho-analysis recognition must be by the sufferer too. The physician considers recognition of the pain subordinate to its cure; the psycho-analyst's view is expressed by Doctor Johnson's letter to Bennet Langton: 'Whether to see life as it is, will give us much consolation, I know not; but the consolation which is drawn from truth, if any there be, is solid and durable; that which may be derived from errour must be, like its original, fallacious and fugitive.'

The point that demonstrates the divergence most clearly is that the physician is dependent on realization of sensuous experience in contrast with the psycho-analyst whose dependence is on experience that is not sensuous. The physician can see and touch and smell. The realizations with which a psycho-analyst deals cannot be seen or touched; anxiety has no shape or colour, smell or sound. For convenience, I propose to use the term 'intuit' as a parallel in the psycho-analyst's domain to the physician's use of 'see', 'touch', 'smell', and 'hear'.

I shall now give three different formulations of the same episode occurring in the psycho-analysis of a woman. More could easily be given to demonstrate the problem of communication and publication that faces the psycho-analyst.

The patient produced an association to express, though in a disguised manner, her hostility to parents whose relationship to each other she represented as that between pander and whore. She intended also to evoke a response from the analyst such that he would be wrong whatever facet of a multi-dimensional association he selected for interpretation. Choice of dimension and interpretation could be 'proved' to reflect the analyst, not the analysand; he could hesitate impotently before the wealth of alternatives presented to him.

A version employing more analytically recondite Kleinian intuitional formulations: the patient was directing an attack on the analyst's psycho-analytic potency; the 'missile' was the association — which therefore is to be

7

regarded as an object of grid category A6. The characteristics of the association are either that it subjects the analyst's intuition to splitting because of his inability to formulate simultaneous expressions of diverse and possibly incompatible interpretations, or that it has the ability to compel the analyst, through the need to act, to adopt a moral standpoint for interpretation because the scientific standpoint involves being 'split' between alternative interpretations. The close relationship between moral attitudes and action, as contrasted with thought or meditation, will be investigated later. The first problem is to choose what interpretation to give. Any one of many facets of the patient's statement may be noticed rather than any other. It can be considered as a statement or as a transformation; as multi-dimensional or multi-faceted; it could be represented by a visual image of a figure in which many planes meet or lines pass through a common point. I can represent it to myself by a visual image of a geometric solid with an infinite number of surfaces. It depends on a realization, derived from space, of sensuous experience. The attempt to externalize the visual image is restricted as if the representation by points and lines was itself a 'space' too restricted to 'contain' the visual image; thus, —— has breadth whereas the *mental* visual image of a line or a point has not.

Projective identification has hitherto been formulated in terms derived from a realization of the ordinary man's (or woman's) idea of three-dimensional space. The usual Kleinian formulations depend on a visual image of a space containing all kinds of objects. Into these objects in this space it is supposed that the patients project parts of their personality that they have split off. Melanie Klein, who discovered this mechanism, considered it to be observable in psychotic and borderline psychotic patients. Later, she and her co-workers considered that the theory had a more extended application and that realizations approximating to it could be detected in neurotic and normal personalities. She stressed the degree of fragmentation and the distance to

8

which the fragments were projected as a determining factor in the degree of mental disturbance the patient displayed in his contact with reality. With this view I agree; as my prac tice with disturbed patients increased it became evident that more rigorous formulation of the theory was needed if the gap between representation and realization was to be bridged by the analyst's interpretation. This was brought home to me in circumstances adumbrated in *Learning from experience* and *Elements of psycho-analysis*. I shall recapitulate briefly some of what I wrote then and later in *Transformations*.

There are patients whose contact with reality presents most difficulty when that reality is their own mental state. For example, a baby discovers its hand; it might as well have discovered its stomach-ache, or its feeling of dread or anxiety, or mental pain. In most ordinary personalities this is true, but people exist who are so intolerant of pain or frustration (or in whom pain or frustration is so intolerable) that they feel the pain but will not suffer it and so cannot be said to discover it. *What* it is that they will not suffer or discover we have to conjecture from what we learn from patients who *do* allow themselves to suffer. The patient who will not suffer pain fails to 'suffer' pleasure and this denies the patient the encouragement he might otherwise receive from accidental or intrinsic relief. Where one patient would understand a word to mark a constant conjunction this patient experiences it as a thing that is not there, and the thing that is not there, like the thing that *is* there, is indistinguishable from an hallucination. Since the term 'hallucination' has a penumbra of associations which would be inappropriate I have named these objects beta-elements.

These descriptions of how these objects appear to the patient and how they appear to me are intended to aid the reader's understanding, but are not sufficiently rigorous for use in practice. The formulations have the status of elements in grid category C.

Suppose the patient is capable of tolerating frustration and pain: his story will differ in important respects from the above. To him the name represents a 'no-thing', but his capacity for toleration enables him to observe a constant conjunction, to bind it with a name or to use it when it has already been named. Patient A, for I shall now call the intolerant patient so, has then at his disposal beta-elements or bizarre objects and his case differs in this respect from patient B, as I now designate the second patient, who can tolerate and therefore name (even if the name is no more than a grunt or a yell) a constant conjunction and so investigate its meaning. Whether the beta-element or the bizarre object is to be classified as thought or not is a matter of scientific convenience which may be determined later. I suggest provisionally that all beta-elements are distinguished from elements that pervade the mental processes of patient B by considering the latter to be thoughts and the former not. The most genetically primitive elements of thought I shall group together as alpha-elements, in distinction to beta-elements.

I shall now use the geometrical concepts of lines, points, and space (as derived originally not from a realization of three-dimensional space but from the realizations of the emotional mental life) as returnable to the realm from which they appear to me to spring. That is, if the geometer's concept of space derives from an experience of 'the place where something was' it is to be returned to illuminate the domain where it is in my experience meaningful to say that 'a feeling of depression' is 'the place where a breast or other lost object was' and that 'space' is 'where depression, or some other emotion, used to be'.

I have pointed out that this space, these points, and these lines differ in one important respect, namely, that in the domain of mental visual images an infinite number of lines may pass through one point but, were I to attempt to represent such a visual image by point and lines on a piece of paper, there would be a finite number of lines. This limiting quality inheres in all realizations of three-dimensional space that approximate to the points, lines, and space of the geometer. It does not inhere in mental space until an attempt is made to represent mental space by verbal thought. I am thus postulating mental space as a thing-in-itself that is unknowable, but that can be represented by thoughts. In thought I include all that is primitive, including alpha-elements as I have so far described them. I exclude, arbitrarily by definition, beta-elements. Thoughts may be classed with the realizations of all objects approximating to the representations of three-dimensional space in this particular: they are intolerable to patient A because they share the frustrating quality of all realizations. Yet to the 'ordinary man' thoughts do not have this restrictive character until it is necessary to apply them to pre-verbal material. Material may be pre-verbal because the individual who seeks to verbalize it has not had sufficient experience of the material to observe a constant conjunction. He is in a state analogous to that seen in a number of similar configurations such as: having pain without suffering it; not understanding planetary movement because the differential calculus has not been invented; not being conscious of a mental phenomenon because it has been repressed; not knowing an event because the event has not occurred.

In all these situations the associated problems require thought for their solution. In all of them thought is restrictive and can be directly experienced as such as soon as an intuition demands representation for private communication. Since thought liberates the intuition there is conflict between the impulse to leave the intuition unexpressed and the impulse to express it. The restrictive element of representation therefore obtrudes in transformation $T\alpha \rightarrow T\beta$ of pre-verbal material. One man achieves the transformation; the other, who cannot tolerate restriction, does not. He therefore forfeits the relief from frustration that thought, were he able to tolerate it, would give. The onset of the reality principle is thus imperilled. In my definition of thought, he will not generate alpha-elements and will not be capable of thought. Whatever substitute he finds for thought is not to be

11

classified as thought. When I discuss psychotic verbalization this point will be considered again.

The failure of alpha-function, which should produce alpha-elements, involves the absence of mental visual images of points, lines, and space. Patient A therefore lacks equipment that would help him to map the realization of mental space. His position is analogous to that of the geometer who had to await the invention of Cartesian co-ordinates before he could elaborate algebraic geometry.

Now consider patient A confronted with an experience in which B would resort to projective identification as adumbrated by Melanie Klein. The restrictive character of reality and the dependence of projective identification on recognition of objects preclude projection of parts of the personality because there is no conception of containers into which the projection could take place. The explosive projection is therefore felt to take place in what is, to the analyst, the *realization* of mental space: a mental space that has no visual images to fulfil the functions of a co-ordinate system, either the 'faceted solid' or the multi-dimensional, multi-linear figure of lines intersecting at a point. The mental realization of space is therefore felt as an immensity so great that it cannot be represented even by astronomical space because it cannot be represented at all.

Paradoxically this explosion is so violent and is accompanied by such immense fear – hereafter referred to as psychotic fear or psychotic panic – that the patient may express it by sudden and complete silence (as if to go to an extreme as far from a devastating explosion as possible).

The ensuing state can be most easily expressed by using surgical shock as a model: in this the dilatation of the capillaries throughout the body so increases the space in which blood can circulate that the patient may bleed to death in his own tissues. Mental space is so vast compared with any realization of three-dimensional space that the patient's capacity for emotion is felt to be lost because emotion itself is felt to drain away and be lost in the immensity. What may then appear to the observer as thoughts, visual images, and verbalizations must be regarded by him as debris, remnants or scraps of imitated speech and histrionic synthetic emotion, floating in a space so vast that its confines, temporal as well as spatial, are without definition. The events of an analysis, spread out over what to the analyst are many years, are to A but the fragments of a moment dispersed in space. The distance in time separating one statement from another can be taken as a measure of the distance in space of one element from another in which all are contemporary. Thus A says he could buy no ice-cream. Six months later he says he cannot even buy ice-cream. Three days later he mentions his being too late to buy ice-cream: there was no ice-cream left. Two years later he says he supposes there was no ice-cream. Had I known, when the topic was mentioned first, what I know now I might have noted the time and place of the reference, but I did not know and therefore could not attend to this statement or note it. When I did, it was because of the obtrusive 'I scream' theme. It was later still that I grasped the significance of 'no − I scream'. By this time, I could make only the vaguest reference to previous appearances of the material. As it turned out this difficulty did not appear to matter and my interpretation was taken. Yet I would feel happier if I thought that my gain in experience could lead to earlier observation and use of the material. I now know that a violent attack had been delivered on a relationship in which the link between the two personalities had been 'I scream'. This had been destroyed and the place of the link 'I scream' had been taken by a 'no − I scream'. The 'I scream' link had itself previously been food, 'ice-cream', a 'breast', until envy and destructiveness had turned the good breast into an 'I scream'. In narrative form: he had been linked to his object by a good breast (he liked ice-cream). This he had attacked, possibly bitten it in actuality. The place of the breast as link was then taken by an 'I scream'. Further attacks made it a 'no −· I scream'. The destruction of the link by explosion now took place in the

13

domain of mental realization. Mental space being infinite, the fragments of the link are dispersed instantaneously over infinite space. The 'distance' between one piece and another is measured in time.[1]

The patient should be shown the evidence on which the interpretation is based; if the evidence is scattered sparsely over a period of years of acting-out, the problem of interpretation assumes serious proportions, because the medium in which the patient is effecting his transformation is not predominantly conversational English, but acting-out. The analysis may be regarded as one moment in time stretched out so that it becomes a line or surface spread out over a period of years – an extremely thin membrane of a moment. Regarded thus, the total analysis can be seen as a transformation in which an intense catastrophic emotional explosion O has occurred (elements of personality, link, and second personality having been instantaneously expelled to vast distances from their point of origin and from each other). This explosive event O is then transformed, in the medium of acting-out and by virtue of beta-elements, to $Tp\beta$, in which space, being restrictive and not amenable to adequate formulation of distance between beta-elements, is replaced by the realization corresponding to time. Though there is no representation of mental space available to the patient and though the realization of three-dimensional space is too restrictive for a temperament intolerant of frustration, the realization of mental space, being unbounded, permits of a continuous and continuing expansion and separation of beta-elements. For the investigation of this mental state the patient cannot, but the analyst can, employ points, lines, and space. The geometer has used them for the investigation of three-dimensional space and, by the substitution of algebraic geometry for the figurative geometry of Euclid, has been

[1] The account I have just given is an example of taking $Tp\beta$ as my TaO, and by $Ta\alpha$ proceeding to $Ta\beta$. $Ta\beta$ is my attempt at a reconstruction of TpO, $Tp\alpha$, $Tp\beta$. When this degree of private communication has been attained, the problem becomes one of publishing it – formulating it in conversational English that the patient can understand (see Bion, 1965).

able to extend his investigation to multi-dimensional space and leave Euclidean space to be used for psychological preparation for the non-Euclidean geometries now available. Can we similarly use the concepts of Euclidean geometry to get back to the emotional realizations from which I believe it originally sprang? The need is for a formulation so general that a multiplication of theories to meet a diversity of realizations bearing the same configuration is obviated, yet so precise that it will not cover configurations whose similarity is only apparent, or whose appearance of similarity is due to irrelevant C category visual imagery.

The impossibility of communication without frustration is so familiar that the nature of the frustration is forgotten. Most people are aware of it as a transient phenomenon experienced on relatively few occasions. In psycho-analytic work the problems are more obtrusive than usual because the subject is novel and its difficulties are uncharted; difficulties become more marked still when the material to be communicated is pre- or non-verbal. The psycho-analyst can employ silences; he, like the painter or musician, can communicate non-verbal material. Similarly, the painter can communicate material that is non-visual and the musician material that is inaudible. The pre-verbal matter the psycho-analyst must discuss is certain to be an illustration of the difficulty in communication that he himself is experiencing. Ability to use points, lines, and space becomes important for understanding 'emotional space', for the continuance of the work and avoidance of a situation in which two inarticulate personalities are unable to release themselves from the bondage of inarticulation. This mutually sterile relationship provides a model for some relationships of the self with itself. When the relationship of the self with itself is of this kind, either the container or the contained must be destroyed. Finally, the individual cannot contain the impulses proper to a pair and the pair cannot contain the impulses proper to a group. The psycho-analytic problem is the problem of growth and its harmonious resolution in the relationship

15

between the container and the contained, repeated in individual, pair, and finally group (intra and extra psychically).

Any definitory hypothesis, be it exclamation, name, theoretical system, or extended statement such as a book, has, and has always been recognized to have, a negative function. It must always imply that something is; equally it implies that something is not. It is therefore open to the recipient to infer one or other according to his temper. If the personality is incapable of tolerating frustration there seems to be no reason why he should not develop on the assumption that the definitory hypothesis means that something is. The statement is then allowed to become a pre-conception and the way is open for the unsaturated element to become saturated. But suppose that the inability to tolerate frustration is 'excessive': the personality may react against the statement, seeing only its negative implications and, in the extreme case, refusing to allow the statement, to him a 'nothing', even to exist. The attempt then is to annihilate the statement in its function of definitory hypothesis. A model would be the infant who cannot tolerate weaning because it is dominated by the *loss* of the breast and who therefore cannot accept what it might have instead. The patient cannot tolerate the definitory hypothesis and therefore does not achieve the pre-conception (D4).

Knowledge of loss, of the negative aspect of the definition, of the 'thought' as a 'no-thing', is immediate; knowledge of gain, if any, has to wait upon the fruits of permitting the thought, or other statement, to be a pre-conception (ψ (ξ)). Therefore 'excessive' inability to tolerate frustration is likely to obstruct development of pre-conception (D4 functions). 'Excessive' intolerance is likely to obstruct awareness of realizations. The 'no-thing' with its corresponding realization (of some object not present) will be liable to destruction whereas 'hallucination' will be favoured for its immediacy. Another formulation of this is to say that the domain of realizations and all that might represent realizations is felt not to afford enough 'space' for freedom whereas the domain of hallucination does. In passing, I must draw attention to the fact that the sense of loss in the definitory hypothesis and the sense of gratification in hallucination both depend on a restricted mental range. In both instances the reaction, of intolerance in one and gratification in the other, might be said to be associated with a short-sighted 'view'. Thought consequently is not seen as offering freedom for development, but is felt as a restriction; by contrast, 'acting-out' is felt to yield a sense of freedom. *A fortiori* an hallucination is designed through its quality as the-thing-itself (not the thought of a breast but the breast itself) to be indistinguishable from freedom. The patient then may be seen as facing a choice: either he may allow his intolerance of frustration to use what might otherwise be a 'no-thing' to become a thought and so achieve the freedom Freud (1911) describes, or he may use what might be a 'no-thing' to be the foundation for a system of hallucinosis.

From this last will spring the set of transformations in hallucinosis which it will be necessary to differentiate from transformations in painting, music, mathematics, and the domain of verbal communication. The importance of making this last distinction is enhanced by the fact that words are used both in the expression of verbal communication and in transformations in hallucinosis. Yet consideration of the nature of the differing reaction to the 'no-thing' will show that the word representing a thought is not the same as the identical word when it is representing an hallucination. Since the similarity may be extremely close in the words employed in both systems and sometimes in the method by which they appear to be combined, it is important to discover in what the difference lies. The difference between philosophy (and even theoretical psycho-analysis) and the practice of psycho-analysis can be seen by considering what the detection of this difference means for the philosopher or theoretician and what it means for the practising psycho-analyst who has to decide in the emotional situation itself whether the patient's statements represent an hallucination or a fact of external reality. It is for this reason that the psycho-analyst must be experienced in non-sensuous realities and able to ignore sensuously derived experience as it appears formalized in memory. The word 'dog' represents different realizations in scientific inquiry and hallucinosis; but the word 'dog' is itself not the same when it is representing a realization in scientific inquiry and an element belonging to the domain of hallucinatory transformations. It is sometimes useful to regard it as analogous to the visual image in a reversible perspective. In the visual image the marks of a drawing on paper remain unchanged but 'mean' two faces or a vase; similarly, 'dog' may mean dog or God (to take but one example). In non-psychotic transformations the invariant is insignificant: the resemblance to ordinary speech, the fact that the word is identical in psychotic and non-psychotic transformation, is accidental.

Verbal, musical, artistic modes of communication all meet with realizations that they appear to represent only very approximately. Hallucination may be regarded, wrongly, as a representation and therefore as unsuited to some activities. As verbal, musical, and artistic transformations have compensating values arising from their being *transformations* of O, it is natural to consider the like possibility with hallucinosis. But hallucinations are *not* representations: they are things-in-themselves born of intolerance of frustration and desire. Their defects are due not to their failure to represent but to their failure to *be*. Thus we need to consider the difference between psychic and external reality.

As I am primarily concerned with the formulation of theory, the illustrations I am about to give are by way of C formulations, not records of clinical experience. The intention is to approach to more rigorous theoretical presentation, that is, presentation less open to misunderstanding through logical defect, or over-flexibility in an attempt to represent different configurations of the same fundamental structures and functions, or failure to represent, through over-rigidity, realizations in which the fundamentals are invariant but the accidentals diverse. The illustrations are C category elements used as preparation for theoretical formulations that can stand by themselves; the reader should regard the 'illustrations' as psychological aids to understanding the theories proper. From this point to the end of the chapter emotional experiences will be represented by C formulations.

1. The patients, for the treatment of whom I wish to formulate theories, experience pain but not suffering. They may be suffering in the eyes of the analyst because the analyst can, and indeed must, suffer. The patient may say he suffers but this is only because he does not know what suffering is and mistakes feeling pain for suffering it. The theory will need to be such that it represents the realization in which this is possible and shows how it comes about. The *intensity* of the patient's pain contributes to his fear of suffering pain.

2. Suffering pain involves respect for the fact of pain, his own or another's. This respect he does not have and therefore he has no respect for any procedure, such as psychoanalysis, which is concerned with the existence of pain.

3. Frustration and intense pain are equated.

4. Pain is sexualized; it is therefore inflicted or accepted but is not suffered – except in the view of the analyst or other observer.

5. For purposes of this exposition the following conjunction is described in narrative form, the elements being sequential and bound in a chain of causation. The realization of the constant conjunction does not have any element that approximates to the sequential or causal elements of the narrative representing it. These features belong only to the C category representation, not to the realization they represent. The patient feels the pain of an absence of fulfilment of his desires. The absent fulfilment is experienced as a 'no-thing'. The emotion aroused by the 'no-thing' is felt as indistinguishable from the 'no-thing'. The emotion is replaced

19

by a 'no-emotion'. In practice this can mean no feeling at all, or an emotion, such as rage, which is a column 2 emotion, that is, an emotion of which the fundamental function is denial of another emotion.

6. As a column 2 element all felt emotion is a 'no-emotion'. In this respect it is analogous to 'past' or 'future' as representing the 'place where the present used to be' before all time was annihilated.

7. The 'place' where time was (or a feeling was, or a 'nothing' of any kind was) is then similarly annihilated. There is thus created a domain of the non-existent. I have not come across any realization that corresponds to such a state though I can imagine a stupor so intense that it might seem to do so. It is nevertheless useful to postulate it partly because there are occasions when it is convenient to suppose that the patient holds such a belief, and partly because it is convenient for the analyst. As will be seen, meanings other than sophisticated meanings creep back into the relatively meaningless state of the term 'non-existent' as E1 category. Some patients with whom I am familiar achieve a state, to which I wish to apply the term 'non-existence', for a few moments at most; this is followed by an externalization or evacuation of 'non-existence'. 'Non-existence' immediately becomes an object that is immensely hostile and filled with murderous envy towards the quality or function of existence wherever it is to be found. 'Space', either as a representation, or the realization the term derives from or represents, becomes terrifying or terror itself: 'Le silence de ces espaces infinies m'effraie.' The space of the ordinary man, the astronomer, or the physicist, becomes confounded with 'mental space', and its objects with the objects of 'mental space'.

8. The scientific or sophisticated approach tends to become confounded with the realizations its formulations are intended to represent. The point (.) and the line (—) are regarded as if they were analogous to representations of

reversible perspective. Their significance therefore varies according to the point of view (or vertex) with which they are associated. Vertices may have as their approximate realizations various recognized disciplines such as religion, mathematics, physics, music, painting, and other arts. The formulations associated with a particular vertex may be categorized in accordance with the grid.

9. The following illustration is to facilitate an approach to a more rigorous representation of 'points of view' or vertices. The patient corresponds to the A personality, the analyst to B. The analytic exchange described is at an advanced stage in the analysis, in the sense that what was an extremely disturbed patient has become better adjusted to what the psycho-analyst regards as reality. The psycho-analyst similarly has become better adjusted to what the patient regards as reality. 'Somewhere' there is present a 'super-ego' that is cruel, denuded of all the characteristics usually associated with the super-ego, and, finally, of 'existence' itself. It therefore has the characteristics of 'non-existence' described in 7 above. I use the term 'super-ego' as a psycho-analytical intuitive theory, now with the status of a realization, which I want to reformulate in terms of another intuitive theory.

The patient talks freely, but his communications are disjointed sentences which would, anywhere but in analysis, be described as 'incoherent'. Such a term is insufficiently illuminating to lead to a psycho-analytical interpretation, but the 'vertex' (the 'point of view' provided by regarding an analysis as an ordinary conversation) gives me a descriptive term suitable for the immediate purpose. As it is not suitable for continuing the psycho-analytic discussion the term 'incoherence' must be observed more critically.

As time passes, and it may require many months of observation, 'incoherence' displays many characteristics and they are changing constantly. The patient may, in a fit of impatience, describe them as pointless; and so they may prove to be, for sentences can indeed communicate everything but the

21

point. The sentences were mutilated. Personal pronouns were used without indication of the person to whom they might relate. Important parts of speech were missing; and so on. The mutilations varied in form and in effect; they did not always make sentences pointless though sometimes 'pointlessness' was the 'point'. This type of peculiarity is but one manifestation of attacks on linking, the technique of psycho-analysis and indeed articulate speech itself being the link. My immediate concern is not with attacks on linking but with an aspect of transformation (Bion, 1965). The patient, having delivered himself of a series of statements, listens to the interpretation and then continues, to all outward appearance, in much the same way. Further observation reveals that there has in fact been a change. If my interpretation was intended to show him that he was speaking to conceal, rather than to reveal, something about his sexual life, he will identify himself with a 'point of view', a vertex, such that only certain elements in my interpretation are illumined. Thus he emulates the mathematician whose formula effects a transformation in vector space. What takes place I shall represent by a slow-motion model:

The patient grasps the gist of what I say. The totality of the statement, including the implication that I am the analyst, is evacuated (the mechanism represented by the theory of projective identification). He identifies himself with the analyst and by virtue of his intuition is able to 'see' the meaning of my interpretation. The meaning that he thus 'sees' is that I am annoyed, jealous, envious at my exclusion from participation in, or understanding of, his sexual life. He then exclaims, 'Oh that frightful noise!'

His remark, without the interpolated story, appears to be a *non sequitur*; if the account given is assumed to represent the mental events, unexpressed in the interval between interpretation and rejoinder, incoherence disappears. Many assumptions can be made about the link between interpretation and response. One set assumes that it should be compatible with respect for the truth; another that it should conform to respect for omniscience; yet another that it should be compatible with both. The role of desire, in pre-conception, is determinant.

In this episode there are some of the unsatisfactory features to which I would draw attention. There is no evidence to support the particular assumption made. To produce it would involve the impossible task of explaining the history of my mental development, or even that limited part of it shared with the patient, that has led to accretions of 'desires' to original beliefs (grid category C1) that my analysand was my patient.

Furthermore, I have used terms, 'omniscient' is one of them, that represent similar developments of meaning in order that the term should become the premiss of further developments. 'Omniscient' is therefore an element categorized as $\overleftarrow{C}3$ and $\overrightarrow{D}4$.

The patient may categorize the same statements in an entirely different way, as is apparent from the description I have given of his interpretation of my interpretation. To meet this difficulty I propose to construct a figure that will serve to represent the invariants of an ever-changing situation.

By way of psychological preparation for the reception of a system that is independent of the particular situations it is intended to serve, I shall use descriptions that lack rigour but have definition. This makes for a lack of flexibility in the final formulation which is intended to combine flexibility with rigour. The system may be regarded as being contained within an emotional space within itself – an 'exo-skeleton' or an 'endo-skeleton'.

To construct this I differentiate an awareness of reality from a denial, or ignoring, or ignorance, of reality. A will ignore reality; B will accept it. With vertex A, reality will be restrictive and frustrating; with vertex B, reality will be liberating and conducive to growth.

Further, I assume an axiomatic approach in all theoretical

formulations; axiomatic statements are not differentiated from postulates and premisses: they are treated as indistinguishable from each other and from definitory hypotheses. Definitory hypotheses are statements marking the binding of a constant conjunction whatever the content of the formulation may be. Any theorem I regard as capable of one of the uses of the horizontal axis. But when a column 1 → columns 3 and 4, it means the category has changed to row D. Any theorem may illuminate facts it was not designed to display, but, conversely, any deductive system will be seen, as soon as it is used, to accumulate meaning in a manner analogous to that of the pre-conception and, in doing so, to require axioms that have not been necessary for the completion of the system.

Any deductive system may appear to be consistent within itself provided it remains definitory, that is to say, with characteristics that qualify it for column 1. The deductions may appear to be consistent and logically necessary so long as it is not asked 'necessary to what?' or 'to whom?' But if they are said to be logically necessary this is itself a statement about the system and this statement cannot be refuted unless it is used. But if it *is* allowed to become saturated, that is to say *used* as a pre-conception, then the pre-conception mates with the realization to produce a conception (E) and again to produce a concept (F). The conception (E) has the characteristic not only that it records by implication (a realization exists which approximates to the pre-conception) but that a realization exists which approximates to the conception although its existence was not known when the pre-conception was formulated. As soon as the deductive system proves its value as an exploratory tool, the self-consistency, which appeared to exist when the domain in which the system applied was limited, is imperilled because readjustments become necessary to fit the theorem to its extended domain. As the system illuminates facts whose significance was unknown before (the elements of the paranoid–schizoid position) and thus imperils its self-consistency, it throws off

24

the limitations of the domain in which it applies. It approximates to illimitability and universality. The dilemma can be stated thus: the system, if consistent within itself, is limited; if not limited, then it cannot be regarded as self-consistent because its self-consistency is contingent. Furthermore, its statements can be seen to depend on an axiomatic statement whose existence was not even suspected, let alone regarded as logically necessary, when the system was formulated and had the status common to column 1 categories.

3 · Reality Sensuous and Psychic

The illustrations in the previous chapter are not satisfactory and I propose to consider some reasons for this.

Psycho-analytical events cannot be stated directly, indubitably, or incorrigibly any more than can those of other scientific research. I shall use the sign O to denote that which is the ultimate reality represented by terms such as ultimate reality, absolute truth, the godhead, the infinite, the thing-in-itself. O does not fall in the domain of knowledge or learning save incidentally; it can be 'become', but it cannot be 'known'. It is darkness and formlessness but it enters the domain K when it has evolved to a point where it can be known, through knowledge gained by experience, and formulated in terms derived from sensuous experience; its existence is conjectured phenomenologically.

The events of the psycho-analytic experience are transformed and formulated. The value of these formulations can be assessed according to the conditions under which the transformations are effected. Formulations of the events of analysis made in the course of analysis must possess value different from that of formulations made extra-sessionally. Their value therapeutically is greater if they are conducive to transformations in O; less if conducive to transformations in K.

The experience of psycho-analysis affords material impossible to equal from any other source. It follows that this material should be available in full to the psycho-analyst. The analysis that every psycho-analyst is obliged to undergo as part of his training is necessary because it removes obstacles to participation in the psycho-analytic experience; it has many facets, but for the psycho-analyst none can compare in importance with this; what I have to say is ancillary to this.

26

It is impossible to undergo an analysis without learning about psycho-analysis as practised by one particular psycho-analyst; this is a misfortune rather than an advantage. Furthermore, established beliefs and conventions, hardened habits of thought, unless subjected to vigilance, re-establish themselves and encroach upon the freedom the psycho-analyst has won by being psycho-analysed and lead to deterioration of his efficiency.

In the course of analysis it is inevitable that the analysand imparts a great deal of information *about* himself just as the analyst imparts information *about* analysis. This information is worthless at best and, at worst, harmful because every analysis is unique; talk about analysis is not.

The analyst must focus his attention on O, the unknown and unknowable. The success of psycho-analysis depends on the maintenance of a psycho-analytic point of view; the point of view is the psycho-analytic vertex; the psycho-analytic vertex is O. With this the analyst cannot be identified: he must *be* it.

Every object known or knowable by man, including himself, must be an evolution of O. It is O when it has evolved sufficiently to be met by K capacities in the psycho-analyst. He does not know the 'ultimate reality' of a chair or anxiety or time or space, but he knows a chair, anxiety, time, and space. In so far as the analyst becomes O he is able to know the events that are *evolutions* of O.

Restating this in terms of psycho-analytic experience, the psycho-analyst can know what the patient says, does, and appears to be, but cannot know the O of which the patient is an evolution: he can only 'be' it. He knows phenomena by virtue of his senses but, since his concern is with O, events must be regarded as possessing either the defects of irrelevancies obstructing, or the merits of pointers initiating, the process of 'becoming' O. Yet interpretations depend on 'becoming' (since he cannot know O). The interpretation is an actual event in an evolution of O that is common to analyst and analysand.

A fallacious but helpful description in A is that the practising analyst must wait for the analytic session to 'evolve'. He must wait not for the analysand to talk or to be silent or to gesture, or for any other occurrence that is an actual event, but for an evolution to take place so that O becomes manifest in K through the emergence of actual events. Similarly, the reader must disregard what I say until the O of the experience of reading has evolved to a point where the actual events of reading issue in his interpretation of the experiences. Too great a regard for what I have written obstructs the process I represent by the terms 'he becomes the O that is common to himself and myself'.

The reasons for this are as follows: There can be no genuine outcome that is based on falsity. Therefore the outcome depends on the closeness with which the interpretative appraisal approximates to truth. The psycho-analyst and his analysand are alike dependent on the senses, but psychic qualities, with which psycho-analysis deals, are not perceived by the senses but, as Freud says, by some mental counterpart of the sense organs, a function that he attributed to consciousness. Without wishing to discard this possibility I prefer to consider it as an open question and substitute a more general postulate which I represent by O. To put it in more popular terms, I would say the more 'real' the psycho-analyst is the more he can be at one with the reality of the patient. Conversely, the more he depends on actual events the more he relies on thinking that depends on a background of sense impression.

In the primitive phase, which Freud regards as dominated by the pleasure principle and from which he excludes the operation of memory, this last being dependent on the prior development of a capacity for thought, the prototype of memory appears to reside in one of the aspects of projective identification. This mechanism, employed to fulfil the duties of thought until thought takes over, appears as an interchange first between mouth and breast and then between introjected mouth and introjected breast. This I regard as reaction between container ♀ and contained ♂. ♀ seems to be the element which is nearest in this phase to the memory. The terms I use must be regarded as verbal representations of visual images; the whole description will be in these C category terms because I find them easier to employ and more likely to be understood. Later, I may attempt more sophisticated formulations.

♂ evacuates unpleasure in order to get rid of it, to have it transformed into something that is, or feels, pleasurable, for the pleasure of evacuation, for the pleasure of being contained. ♀ takes in the evacuations for the same motives. The nature of the relationship needs investigation. ♀, which may evacuate or retain, is the prototype of a forgetful or retentive memory. Pleasure may be retained if possession is the dominant concern; grievance if a store of ammunition is the main concern. Evacuation may be forcible as if to convert the evacuated object into a missile; introjection likewise as fulfilment of greed. Developments of memory that are inevitable to the psycho-analyst are C category elements, the dominance of ♀♂, the primacy of pleasure–pain (in contrast with reality or truth), and 'possession' with its reciprocal, fear of loss; all have been acquired in close association with the senses.

The impulse to be rid of painful stimuli gives the 'content' of the memory (♀) an unsatisfactory quality when one is engaged in the pursuit of truth O. The more successful the memory is in its accumulations the more nearly it approximates to resembling a saturated element saturated with saturated elements. An analyst with such a mind is one who is incapable of learning because he is satisfied. Furthermore, because of its primitive nature, his memory is believed to be filled only with objects giving rise to feelings of pleasure and to be empty of unpleasure components, or vice versa. The attitude towards the 'memory' or 'unconscious' depends on the idea that it is a container for the 'evacuations' of projective identification. Such a 'memory' is no equipment for an analyst whose aim is O, as may be seen by considering what is represented by this sign.

It stands for the absolute truth in and of any object; it is assumed that this cannot be known by any human being; it can be known about, its presence can be recognized and felt, but it cannot be known. It is possible to be at one with it. That it exists is an essential postulate of science but it cannot be scientifically discovered. No psycho-analytic discovery is possible without recognition of its existence, at-one-ment with it and evolution. The religious mystics have probably approximated most closely to expression of experience of it. Its existence is as essential to science as to religion. Conversely, the scientific approach is as essential to religion as it is to science and is as ineffectual until a transformation from K → O takes place.

In order to know about the analysand the analyst has recourse to K. Memory is a part of K. Notation (Freud, 1911), in the wide sense of the term, is its servant. But memory depends on the senses. It is limited by the limitations of the senses and their subordination to the pleasure–pain principle; memories are therefore fallacious and memory has the defects of its origin in functions of possessiveness and evacuation.

The psycho-analyst is concerned with O, which is incommunicable save through K activity. O may appear to be attainable by K through phenomena, but in fact that is not so. K depends on the evolution of O → K. At-one-ment with O would seem to be possible through the transformation K → O, but it is not so. The transformation O → K depends on ridding K of memory and desire. I turn accordingly to consider 'desire'.

It may not seem necessary to postulate desire as well as memory: if memory could be dispensed with, desire would likewise disappear and vice versa. But this would involve loss of meaning which I wish to retain. So, in addition to memories, I wish to consider thoughts, which are formulations of desire, and probably, but not certainly, objects we represent by the term 'desire'. They are not verbal formulations merely, or even verbal formulations of elements of C

30

category. The desires that can be represented verbally are relatively simple to deal with. For example, the thought occurs that one would like to go abroad for the annual holiday; this can be followed by further ideas, more or less detailed elaborations of the main theme. These thoughts are typical 'desires'; they are extremely common and can be harboured almost unaware; they may be reminiscences or anticipations.

The 'memories' and 'desires' to which I wish to draw attention have the following elements in common: they are ready formulated and therefore require no formulation; they derive from experience gained through the senses; they are evocations of feelings of pleasure or pain; they are formulations 'containing' pleasure or pain. In so far as they are column 2 statements their function is to prevent transformation of the K → O order.

The above characteristics cannot be indulged by the psycho-analyst without impairment of analytic capacity. For any who have been used to remembering what patients say and to desiring their welfare, it will be hard to entertain the harm to analytic intuition that is inseparable from *any* memories and *any* desires.

The first point is for the analyst to impose on himself a positive discipline of eschewing memory and desire. I do not mean that 'forgetting' is enough: what is required is a positive act of refraining from memory and desire.

It may be wondered what state of mind is welcome if desires and memories are not. A term that would express approximately what I need to express is 'faith' — faith that there is an ultimate reality and truth — the unknown, unknowable, 'formless infinite'. This must be believed of every object of which the personality can be aware: the evolution of ultimate reality (signified by O) has issued in objects of which the individual can be aware. The objects of awareness are aspects of the 'evolved' O and are such that the sensuously derived mental functions are adequate to apprehend them. For them faith is not required; for O it is. The analyst is not concerned with such sensuously apprehended

31

objects or with knowledge of such objects. Memories and desires are worthless but inevitable features that he encounters in himself as he works. He *is* concerned with these objects in his analysand because he is concerned with the working of the analysand's mind. His analysand will express his awareness of O in people and things by formulations representing the intersection of evolutions of O with the evolution of his awareness.

It is not possible to say that such formulations by the analysand are not to be interpreted: no such rule can be laid down far from the situation in which it is to be applied because the criteria for it do not exist. Nor can the criteria be established in the situation of the analysis, for they are part of an ineffable experience. There can be no rules about the nature of the emotional experience that will show that the emotional experience is ripe for interpretation. Instead I can only suggest rules for the analyst that will help him to achieve the frame of mind in which he is receptive to O of the analytic experience. If he is able to be receptive to O, then he may feel impelled to deal with the intersection of the evolution of O with the domain of objects of sense or of formulations based on the senses. Whether he does so or not cannot depend on *rules* for O, or O → K, but only on his ability to be at one with O.

My last sentence represents an 'act' of what I have called 'faith'. It is in my view a scientific statement because for me 'faith' is a scientific state of mind and should be recognized as such. But it must be 'faith' unstained by any element of memory or desire. If it reveals an aspect of O which has to be formulated, then the *transformation* will require the operation of memory and desire; even so the formulation will require the negative characteristics of column 1 elements – that is to say that the statements must affirm implicitly that the object defined is *not* any of the elements whose names are used in the definitory hypothesis, but is a constant conjunction whose meaning will declare itself only when all traces of memory and desire have been removed from the elements invoked to produce the new formulation. Failure to observe the nature of transformation O → K (that is, the use of objects of memory and desire to mark a new constant conjunction, and the need to discard the evocative characteristics of memory and desire so that the formulation representing the new constant conjunction is unsaturated) has obscured the only sense in which the term 'abstraction' has any useful meaning. A formulation has the quality of an abstraction only in so far as it is divorced from the sensuous background inherent in and essential to memory and desire. The abstract statement must not stimulate memory and desire though memory and desire have contributed elements to its formulation.

Memory and desire are essential elements in the composition of the new formulation, but a distinction must be made between two classes of mental event. One is an evocation of memory and desire with impulses of possessiveness and sensuous greed: the impulses generate memory and desire; memory and desire generate sensuous greed. The other is the evocation of memories and desires because the experience of at-one-ment *resembles* possession and sensuous fulfilment. The classes differ because the mode of selection differs, and since the classes differ the interpretation (the formulation by the analyst) will differ. The evocation of that which provided a container for possessions, and of the sensuous gratifications with which to fill it, will differ from an evocation stimulated by at-one-ment. The· exercises in discarding memory and desire must be seen as preparatory to a state of mind in which O can evolve. The facilitation of 'constellation'[1] must in turn be seen as a step in the process of at-one-ment (the transformation O → K). In practice this means not that the analyst recalls some relevant memory but that a relevant constellation will be evoked during the process of at-one-ment with O, the process denoted by transformation O → K.

[1] I use the term 'constellation' to represent the process precipitating a constant conjunction.

33

To what then *is* the analyst's memory relevant and why can there not be a constellation that has a relevance other than relevance to analysis?

It is difficult to conceive of an analysis having a satisfactory outcome without the analysand's becoming reconciled to, or at one with, himself. It is tempting to suppose that such an outcome, or the desire for such an outcome, might provide a criterion for relevance. Conversely, it would be convenient if the analyst's memories, as reminiscences of sensuous experience, could be disregarded as column 2 phenomena mobilized to keep at bay the experience inseparable from the transformations in O. If the objection to memory can be sustained because all memory is a special case of keeping (possessing) a theory known to be (or suspected of being) false in order to prevent the psychological upheaval inseparable from mental growth, it will have the advantage of decreasing the number of theories required to extend, as I propose to do, the theories of resistance. It is sometimes said that a particular interpretation is inadvisable because it increases resistances, but any approach produces its proper resistances and it is as possible to identify an approach by its resistances as it is to judge a tree by its fruit. Resistance to growth is endo-psychic and endo-gregious; it is associated with turbulence in the individual and in the group to which the growing individual belongs.

C category elements, developed from experience gained by the senses, all have gratificatory quality associated with dominance of the pleasure–pain principle. Objections to 'memories' and 'desires' are therefore objections to C3 and C3(2) statements. Later it will be necessary when we deal with hallucinations to distinguish between C elements having a background of visual sensation and those with other sense backgrounds.

The discipline that I propose for the analyst, namely avoidance of memory and desire, in the sense in which I have used those terms, increases his ability to exercise 'acts of faith'. An 'act of faith' is peculiar to scientific procedure

34

and must be distinguished from the religious meaning with which it is invested in conversational usage; it becomes apprehensible when it can be represented in and by thought. It must 'evolve' before it can be apprehended and it is apprehended when it is a thought just as the artist's O is apprehensible when it has been transformed into a work of art. But the 'act of faith' is not a statement, not even a column 6 statement, though it has resemblances to column 6 elements. All grid elements have a background of O from which they have evolved and it is only when O has evolved sufficiently to be apprehended that it can be represented by a grid element. It is only when it has evolved to the point where it can be represented by a grid element that it can be apprehended. When it is apprehended the element can be represented by a grid category.

The 'act of faith' has no association with memory or desire or sensation. It has a relationship to thought analogous to the relationship of *a priori* knowledge to knowledge. It does not belong to the $\pm K$ system but to the O system. It does not by itself lead to knowledge 'about' something, but knowledge 'about' something may be the outcome of a defence against the consequences of an 'act of faith'. A thought has as its realization a no-thing. An 'act of faith' has as its background something that is unconscious and unknown because it has not happened. Thoughts have as their background realizations that are sensible: anxiety, fear, sex can be thought about only when O has evolved to a point where it is apprehensible in sense and has become amenable to transformations in K. Anxiety is 'known' by its secondary qualities. Yet no one has any doubt about anxiety or about 'feeling' the reality, though what is felt is sensations associated with anxiety and not anxiety itself. Similarly, no one who denudes himself of memory and desire, and of all those elements of sense impression ordinarily present, can have any doubt of the reality of the psycho-analytical experience which remains ineffable.

Receptiveness achieved by denudation of memory and

desire (which is essential to the operation of 'acts of faith') is essential to the operation of psycho-analysis and other scientific proceedings. It is essential for experiencing hallucination or the state of hallucinosis.

This state I do not regard as an exaggeration of a pathological or even natural condition: I consider it rather to be a state always present, but overlaid by other phenomena, which screen it. If these other elements can be moderated or suspended hallucinosis becomes demonstrable; its full depth and richness are accessible only to 'acts of faith'. Elements of hallucinosis of which it is possible to be sensible are the grosser manifestations and are of secondary importance; to appreciate hallucination the analyst must participate in the state of hallucinosis. From what I have said it will be clear that this is so, for I have postulated that a K link can operate only on a background of the senses, is capable of yielding only knowledge 'about' something, and must be differentiated from the O link essential to transformations in O. Before interpretations of hallucination can be given, which are themselves transformations O → K, it is necessary that the analyst undergoes in his own personality the transformation O → K. By eschewing memories, desires, and the operations of memory he can approach the domain of hallucinosis and of the 'acts of faith' by which alone he can become at one with his patients' hallucinations and so effect transformations O → K.

A type of hallucination worthy of study is that which one may describe provisionally as visual. I have described a patient who seemed to think that my words flew over his head and could be detected in what to me were the patterns on a cushion. I have since found that the pattern on the cushion was seen by him to travel, as it were, in the opposite direction. That is, he was able, in a state of hallucinosis, to see that the patterns were really my words travelling, through his eyes, to him. Furthermore the 'meaning', which could not be grasped outside the conditions of hallucinosis, was perfectly clear in a state of hallucinosis. The 'meaning' of a statement in hallucinosis is not, however, the same as its meaning in the domain of rational thought. Ordinarily, constellation, constant conjunction, and binding (by nomenation) are a prelude to exploration of meaning. In the domain of hallucinosis the mental event is transformed into a sense impression and sense impressions in this domain do not have meaning; they provide pleasure or pain. In this way the unsense-able mental phenomenon is transformed into a beta-element which can be evacuated and reintroduced so that the act yields, not a meaning, but pleasure or pain.

The analysand in a state of hallucinosis experiences visual hallucinations which tend to be self-perpetuating. They yield pleasure and pain, both being valued, and fail to yield meaning in the sense in which that term is understood in the domain of rational thought. He tends therefore to demand, and provide, more hallucination to compensate for the missing gratification. He feels the pleasure and pain to be inadequate; the 'meaning' is likewise inadequate. The less gratification he achieves the more greedy he becomes; the more greedy, the more hallucinated. The visual element is expected to be exempt from the disabilities inherent in those senses that depend for their efficacy on proximity to the object of gratification. Meaning is lost, pain and pleasure are gained, from a state that is independent of proximity to an object and of the frustration peculiar to thoughts and their genetic association with the 'no-thing'.[1]

I suspect that what I have said of visual hallucinations is true of hallucinations with a background of senses other than visual, but other senses lack the quality of independence of close contact with objects.

A patient who feared guilt substituted punishment. It was achieved by hallucinosis. His circumstances were comfortable and he did not manipulate events by acting out, which he might have done, to produce a penitential life. He could

[1] It is worth contrasting this type of independence of objects, conferred by hallucinosis and the advantages of 'visual' impression, with the independence of the physical presence of objects peculiar to 'maths' and 'thinking'. Note, too, the distraction caused by the *presence* of objects.

presumably have forced the police to take action by committing some variety of sexual offence – sexual offences often appeared in his statements – but instead he complained incessantly though inarticulately of what he ultimately came to recognize as sexual visions, which he admitted were present throughout the sessions. For months during which I had interpreted that he was seeing visions he denied them, but they were maintained tenaciously. After their presence had been admitted he feared to lose them though their dominance was painful. The pain yielded pleasure, and therefore there was cause for him to cherish the state of which he complained. His complaints, his flow of statements, produced a painful state in analysis and then were made into a sexual link between him and me. At the stage of which I write this was a gratification and also a protection against behaviour which might yield pleasure in a more expansive way – by his becoming involved with the police, for example. But his fear of any change was so acute that it was impossible to say with any plausibility what he expected to take the place of his hallucinations were they to cease. In time, however, certain fears could be discussed. Acting-out limited the amount of experience and its extent because the reality component involved frustration and delay, and real pain and pleasure seemed deficient in power to satisfy.[1] This, however, was his complaint against hallucinatory gratification. Hallucinations of dreams seemed to be deficient in associations and unsuited to perform the functions of dreams, and to be felt as unrewarding. Yet he reported what he said were dreams.

In this period hallucination supplied him with punishment as it might in other circumstances have supplied him with sexual pleasure, food, or any other sensual gratification. His analysis indeed showed that the usefulness of hallucination was absolutely limited to elements with a background of sense-able realizations: this was their virtue and their defect.

[1] In this respect real objects, real pain and pleasure, are felt as distraction. It is worth comparing *this* type of distraction with the frustration experienced by a calculator who has to think out mathematical problems only in the presence of objects which are the essence of his calculation.

Their moral value seemed to be that they punished him by providing him with ill-deserved pain to compensate for having been once used as the source of ill-deserved pleasure. In the analytic session they seemed as a barrier against any appreciation of the realities of the session. Yet some interpretations were grasped sometimes. I found it difficult to establish any rule that would govern the time at which interpretations could be understood but I did note that the interpretation had to be exact. He could not correct or adjust an inexactitude so as to bring the interpretation into line with the realization it was intended to illumine. It had to remain uncorrected and unabsorbed because it was wrong.

The sessions were occupied in verbalization of his visual images. His verbalizations were peppered with locutions such as 'tomorrow', 'yesterday', 'last week', all of which could be taken to mean 'not now'. Splitting in time was very common and psycho-analytic objects were scattered over a range of years. Corresponding to this was a denial of the present which amounted to a denial of the passage of time. It was as if a moment of time had been stretched out to cover an enormous area as if it were a piece of elastic.

There had been an occasion when he smelled coffee in the house where I was working. He had once seen me caught in a rain shower without a coat or umbrella. Both these facts appeared in fragments spread out over many years. It would be an exaggeration to say they were expressed unmistakably. I have no doubt, or, more accurately, by an 'act of faith' I am confident, that the scraps of sentences and intonations when put together were signs that he had had both these experiences as I have described them. Were it possible for him to witness my having coffee and being caught in the rain, to 'take it in' and then fragment what he had thus taken in, to evacuate these fragments and leave them scattered over a wide space of time, then that would be what he was doing. The two facts appear in the analysis as if they have been embedded in the elastic moment of time that has been stretched out to cover an enormous area. How far is it safe to use such descriptions as a valid basis for conjecture? I can imagine that this patient's grasp of fact is so slight that he has not enough with which to provide a cover for his psychotic mechanisms. Further, I can suppose that the obtrusion of psychotic mechanisms is such that the 'skin' or 'sanity' is stretched to breaking-point. Either description is likely to be so limited as to lead to a multiplicity of theories to serve a single configuration. But an illumination for the psycho-analyst does not necessarily provide illumination for someone not sharing the experience or illuminate for the patient who shares the experience but who transforms it under hallucinosis.

This problem prompts comparison of interpretation with the matter interpreted, or comparison of the category of associations with the category of the interpretation; the grid is an instrument by which this can be effected. If some relationship between the categories could be established it might be possible to discover the nature of the relationship between psychotic association and the appropriate interpretation. This involves a further look at projective transformation.

The views expressed about memory and desire and the need for their regulation as the psycho-analyst's preparation for his work provide a starting-point for reconsidering the nature of the projective transformation. Hallucinosis, which can be *observed* by divesting oneself of memory and desire, must have had some corresponding mechanism in the events that led to its inception. If the analyst can take certain steps that enable him to 'see' what the patient sees, it is reasonable to suppose that the patient has likewise 'taken steps', though not necessarily the same ones, to enable him to 'see' what he sees.

4 · Opacity of Memory and Desire

The 'act of faith' (*F*) depends on disciplined denial of memory and desire. A bad memory is not enough: what is ordinarily called forgetting is as bad as remembering. It is necessary to inhibit dwelling on memories and desires. They are two facets of the same thing: both are composed of elements based on sense impressions; both imply the absence of immediate sensual satisfaction; one supposes a store of sensual objects, the memory being the container, and the other a conjunction of sensually satisfying objects. The invariants are an inside and an outside composed of objects which are sensible. The more the psycho-analyst occupies himself with memory and desire the more his facility for harbouring them increases and the nearer he comes to undermining his capacity for F. For consider: if his mind is preoccupied with what is or is not said, or with what he does or does not hope, it must mean that he cannot allow the experience to obtrude, particularly that aspect of it which is more than the sound of the patient's voice or the sight of his postures. What sounds the patient makes, or what spectacle he presents, relates to O only in so far as O has evolved into the K domain.

Uninhibited exercise of memories and desires is indistinguishable from, inseparable from, and analogous to, making pre-conception impossible by virtue of leaving no unsaturated element (the desire or the memory precludes pre-conception if it occupies the 'space' that should remain unsaturated). If the mind is preoccupied with elements perceptible to sense it will be that much less able to perceive elements that cannot be sensed. Yet obviously anxiety cannot be said, except by analogy, to be smelled or touched or felt. Even so, anxiety comes nearer to being 'sensed' than

41

many more subtle aspects of the personality which do nevertheless exist. It is important that the analyst should avoid mental activity, memory and desire, which is as harmful to his mental fitness as some forms of physical activity are to physical fitness.

'Past' and 'future' represent a realization related to another realization represented by the terms 'internal' and 'external'. The past is something contained 'within' the 'memory', and the 'future' something that cannot be so contained. 'Memories' can be regarded as possessions; desires, though just as much 'in' the mind as are memories, and therefore just as much 'possessions', are spoken of as if they 'possessed' the mind. A certain class of patient feels 'possessed' by or imprisoned 'in' the mind of the analyst if he considers the analyst desires something relative to him – his presence, or his cure, or his welfare. I have said if the patient 'considers' the analyst desires something, but in fact to say in this context that the patient 'considers' is to use an approximation that may be misleading because its penumbra of association conceals more than it reveals of the state of mind of the patient. The patient is in a state of mind for which there is no verbal apparatus and the psycho-analyst is constantly faced by the need to produce his own apparatus for investigation while he is carrying on the investigation. If the psycho-analyst has not deliberately divested himself of memory and desire the patient can 'feel' this and is dominated by the 'feeling' that he is possessed by and contained in the analyst's state of mind, namely, the state represented by the term 'desire'.

A means of representing mental phenomena without words (which are unsuitable because of their background of sensible experience) is required. The patient uses words that represent visual images, or he may be mute for long periods, or use words that are evocations of emotion, sometimes powerful emotions, but challenge the psycho-analyst to detect a content and express it in ordinary English. Evocations of anger, anxiety, fear, pity, hate, and loyalty to himself often include words that give the total a particular coloration: wreath, upset, cemetery, may be words scattered through the flow in such a way as to suggest bereavement; or solicitors, damages, illness, to suggest legal proceedings. In this way he appears to be having an experience that he is not able to represent in terms of ordinary speech. He could be described therefore as suffering from a speech disorder were it not that the disturbance would appear to be inadequately or eccentrically described in such terms; reciprocally, to ordinary view, it seems eccentric to say that a stammerer suffers from a psychosis. But in fact the descriptions of the psychotic patient as having a speech disorder and the stammerer as being psychotic both have substance, and in both eccentricity depends on the vertex. 'Stammer' and 'psychosis' are vertices displaying the same configuration in a manner that illuminates characteristics just as binocular vision demonstrates qualities that require stereoscopy to make them manifest.

Freud, in a letter to Lou Andreas-Salome, suggested his method of achieving a state of mind which would give advantages that would compensate for obscurity when the object investigated was peculiarly obscure. He speaks of blinding himself artificially. As a method of achieving this artificial blinding I have indicated the importance of eschewing memory and desire. Continuing and extending the process, I include understanding and sense perception with the properties to be eschewed. The suspension of memory, desire, understanding, and sense impressions may seem to be impossible without a complete denial of reality; but the psycho-analyst is seeking something that differs from what is normally known as reality; a criticism that applies to what is ordinarily meant by reality does not indicate undesirability for the purpose of achieving contact with psychic reality, namely, the evolved characteristics of O. This procedure is valid in psycho-analysis and other sciences; F, likewise, is an essential component of scientific procedure however rigorous.

43

There is the possibility of suppressing one or all of these functions of memory, desire, understanding, and sense either together or in turn. Practice in suppression of these faculties may lead to an ability to suppress one or other according to need, so that suspension of one might enhance the effect of domination by the other in a manner analogous to the use of alternate eyes.

Before considering the distinction to be made between total suppression, sleep or other recognized states we must consider in more detail what is meant by understanding or memory or desire. I accept Freud's view of memory and its relationship with notation (Freud, 1911). Since all memory has a background of sense impressions, the appropriate category is row C. As there are a number of respects in which memory and desire seem to have a similar configuration I propose to consider only the C3 function of memory. What of a 'memory' of a gratification that was *missed*? – an unfulfilled desire must be classed as a desire.[1] If the constellation of thought to which it belongs is associated with feelings of grievance, regret, or remorse, such a desire may have to be regarded by the psycho-analyst as dominating or possessing the memory. A practising psycho-analyst has to decide whether he is psycho-analytically witnessing the operation of a *particular* internal object or not. Does the patient feel like that, or does what he feels like approximate to the formulations of Melanie Klein? I am concerned with developing a mode of thought which is such that a correct clinical observation can be made, for if *that* is achieved there is always hope of evolution of the appropriate theory. Defective observation means that a correct interpretation is an accident. The memory can become possessed by a desire; it can cease to be felt as a possession but itself becomes a possessor of the personality that harbours it. The category is no longer C3. What then is it? The unwelcome answer is that so long as progress, growth, is taking place, no one knows.

The probability is that either a process of rationalization

[1] To be a desire the idea must be felt to be unfulfilled.

leads to its conversion to categories D → F and columns 2, 4, 5, 6, n − 1, n 1, or it becomes fixed in row C and column 2. The need to resist the impact of changing circumstances requires that the C2 memory should become more and more independent of, and impervious to, the world of reality (sensible). These are developments in the category C3(2) and are, according to intensity, memories of sense impressions designed to act as a barrier *against* sense impressions; it would seem likely to lead to a development akin to hallucinations. The solution of the problem is made nearer by giving 'projective identification' a direction and greatly increasing the vertices and destinations. Not enough attention is paid to the unconscious as itself a destination of the projected object nor yet to the evacuation from the mental world into the sensible world and so out of the mental system.

Desire is similar to memory in that both have a background of sense impressions. But desire relates to that which is felt not to be possessed; it is 'unsaturated'. There is therefore a correspondence between desire as an unsaturated term and the evolution of O it represents. The problem in discussing O is that the discussion can only be about evolved characteristics of O (K) whereas F is related to O itself.

The problem of differentiating desire from memory lies in the fact that it is 'located' in a 'place' which cannot be determined any more than can the 'place' where parallel lines of a railway-track meet. 'Where' is a term with a background of sense impressions. The difference between desire and memory has no background of sense impressions and cannot be discussed adequately in terms that have such a background. Nevertheless, in psycho-analytic practice it is possible to decide when memory is being experienced by the patient and when desire: one is the 'past' tense and the other the 'future'. The decision depends on the fact that the experience the analyst has of the patient's experience is different from the patient's experience. Investigation of the problems involved depends on F. This means that the understanding of

45

the patient and the identification with him that have been regarded as sufficient hitherto must be replaced by something quite different. The transformation in K must be replaced by the transformation in O, and K must be replaced by F. Now in transformations in K, the point on which attention is focused lies on the line of intersection of the evolution of O with Tα to produce Tβ. In transformation in O, the attention is focused beyond the intersection and in O. Tα and Tβ are therefore projections onto a surface from a point at O (infinity), and although O (infinity) is inaccessible to K it is perfectly accessible to T in O. The analyst has to *become infinite* by the suspension of memory, desire, understanding. The emotional state of transformations in O is akin to dread as it is represented by the formulation:

> *Like one that on a lonesome road*
> *Doth walk in fear and dread;*
> *And having once turned round walks on,*
> *And turns no more his head;*
> *Because he knows a frightful fiend*
> *Doth close behind him tread.*

The 'frightful fiend' represents indifferently the quest for truth or the active defences against it, depending on the vertex.

The menace to 'reality' is felt to derive from: (1) the suppression of memory, desire, and understanding, for such suppression undermines sense-based experience which is the reality with which the individual is familiar; (2) the increase of power of F, which reveals and makes possible experiences that are often painful and difficult for the individual analyst and analysand to tolerate; and (3) the peculiar type of relationship between one element and another in the O domain. Included in this is a relationship that is indifferently expressed as spatial or temporal. Thus, in my quotation, the walker is being 'overtaken' by dread; he walks a 'lonesome road'. It may seem improbable that dread should be associated with analytic progress towards a more realistic outlook. I shall therefore discuss the phenomenon at greater length.

First it is to be noted that the submergence of memory, desire, and understanding appears not only to run flat contrary to accepted procedure but also to be close to what occurs spontaneously in the severely regressed patient.[1] The analyst who tries this disciplinary activity will find it disturbing despite his own analysis, however thorough and prolonged it might have been. It is necessary to consider why this should be so.

Desire, memory, and understanding are based on sensuous experience, expressed in terms whose background is precisely the same experience and which are designed for use related to that experience. They are vitiated by the same defect as are formulations based on a background of inanimate reality when they are applied to biological reality. Anxiety, depression, persecution are not *sensed* (though common usage sanctions an analogical use of the term 'sensed' in a context in which it is not appropriate). The nearer the analyst comes to achieving suppression of desire, memory, and understanding, the more likely he is to slip into a sleep akin to stupor. Though different, the difference is hard to define. The sharpening of contact with O cannot be separated from an increase of perception, in particular of elements of K; this sensuous sharpening is painful although partial and mitigated by the general obliteration of sensory perception. The residual sensory perception, often auditory and restricted to particular kinds of sound, is responsible for inducing a sharp and painful reaction (similar to the startle reaction seen in babies).

Furthermore, the sacrifice of pleasure and pain is a deprivation that is not easily tolerated in prospect and is disliked by the analysand when he senses it in the analyst. The deprivation corresponds to displacement of the pleasure–

[1] There are real dangers associated with the appearance; this is why the procedure here adumbrated is advocated only for the psycho-analyst whose own analysis has been carried at least far enough for the recognition of paranoid–schizoid and depressive positions.

pain principle from its dominant position. This would not matter were it not for a simultaneous apparent deposition of the reality principle, for that is based on a background of realizations which are perceptible to the psyche through the mediation of the senses. The disciplined increase of F by suppression of K, or subordination of transformations in K to transformations in O, is therefore felt as a very serious attack on the ego until F has become established. If psycho-analytic method is narrowly conceived of as consisting in the accumulation of knowledge (possessiveness), in harmony with the reality principle, and divorced from the processes of maturation and growth (either because growth is not recognized or because it is recognized but felt to be unattainable and beyond the control of the individual), it becomes a potent stimulus of envy. A further source of distortion is the tendency to link F with the supernatural because of lack of experience of the 'natural' to which it relates. The tendency is to introduce a god or devil that F is to reveal (or that is to 'evolve' from O). The element F, which should remain un-saturated, becomes saturated and unfitted for its purpose. The progressive stages in the disciplinary exercise proposed for the analyst are repellent rather than attractive. The more the analyst becomes expert in excluding memory, desire, and understanding from his mental activity, the more he is likely, at least in the early stages, to experience painful emotions that are usually excluded or screened by the conventional apparatus of 'memory' of the session, analytical theories, often disguised desires or denials of ignorance, and 'understanding' (which consists more often than not of column 2 elements). I exclude consideration of painful ex-periences in so far as they lie in unresolved conflicts in the ana-lyst, for these do not differ from similar experiences in the practice of accepted methods; I have nothing to add to what is already known of counter-transference and the complica-tions to which it may give rise. But it may be as well to glance at some of the more common experiences if only as a warning to anyone disposed to practise the approach I advocate.

In the first place, the analyst will soon find that he appears to be ignorant of knowledge which he has hitherto regarded as the hallmark of scrupulous medical responsibility. It is disconcerting to find that one is without an idea, say, that the patient has been married, or has children, or of certain events deemed by the analysand to have been of great significance. If the patient has paranoid trends and displays a tendency towards litigation it may seem to be running an unwarranted risk to be ignorant of matters that could, in a court of law, be regarded as significant and as evidence of ordinary medical care for detail. This would indeed be the case if there were not cogent reasons for *not* 'remembering' such detail. As it is, I think that whatever the risks may be the obligation is for the analyst to conduct the case in accordance with his lights – and not in accordance with the supposed risks to himself. In this method the experience the analyst gains bears little resemblance to the files and case-histories with which psychiatry is familiar. It may appear to differ from what would be expected in the light of accepted analytic theory. Thus an analyst may feel, to take a common example, that his married patient is unmarried; if so, it means that psycho-analytically his patient *is* unmarried: the emotional reality and the reality based on the supposition of the marriage contract are discrepant. If this seems to suggest the analyst must preserve his capacity for memory, I maintain that he always does (as does the patient, however regressed), but error is more likely to arise through inability to *divest* oneself of memory than through forgetfulness. If the analyst does not remember that his patient is married, the fact that he *is* is irrelevant until the patient says something that reminds the analyst of this fact.

I have spoken of the 'fact' that the patient is married. Sooner or later it will be necessary to abandon locutions which, though helpful when adumbrated (i.e. used to bind a constant conjunction), become unable to fulfil the function for which they are intended. To take the present instance as an example: provided one does not consider too deeply what

49

is meant, no difficulty is experienced in using the phrase, or the idea that is represented by the phrase, 'the patient is married'. But in psycho-analysis such matters as the patient's marriage have to be considered deeply. Is an overt practising homosexual with several children and a wife with whom he has entered into the marriage contract married? In psycho-analysis the answer does not depend only on what is meant by marriage, because marriage is but one 'element' among many: for example, the 'meaning' of having several children, or a wife or husband with whom a legal marriage has been contracted. In such a context the value can be seen of regarding both the term 'marriage' (the verbal expression) and the fact of several children, and a wife or husband, as 'statements' whose grid category can be determined. If one considers the 'fact' of marriage it soon becomes necessary to suppose a number of different kinds of fact, such as a fact of 'external reality' or a fact of 'psychic reality'. Such terms are useful but they are themselves statements, and the belief that an event belongs to a category of 'events of external reality' leads to confusion and contradiction. It is simpler to regard the patient's statements as having a category in the vertex of the analyst and to observe that they do not, in the analyst's view, 'mean' that the patient is married (i.e. they are not column 3 elements) but that they have a particular category and that it is from the analyst's assessment of the category that the 'meaning' derives. *His* unsaturated elements are saturated. What the patient *thinks* he means is, as far as the analyst is concerned, irrelevant, but what the statement *is*, and to what use it is put, *is* relevant. What matters is that to statements of a particular category the patient begins to add statements of a different category. The patient whose statements have at no time suggested to the analyst that he, the patient, is married, now, at a particular point in his analysis, introduces statements that indicate that he *is*; that is to say, he behaves in a way that makes the analyst regard his statements as belonging to new categories including column 6 (he is asserting that he has actually *done* something, resorted to

50

the kind of statement that consists in actually doing something, e.g. getting married).

Now it is clear that if the psycho-analyst has allowed himself the unfettered play of memory, desire, and understanding, his pre-conceptions will be habitually saturated and his 'habits' will lead him to resort to instantaneous and well-practised saturation from 'meaning' rather than from O. When the psycho-analyst anticipates some crisis, and especially if he has, or thinks he has, good grounds for anxiety, his tendency is to resort to memory and understanding to satisfy his desire for security (or to resort to 'saturation' to avoid 'unsaturation'). If he gives in to this tendency he is proceeding in a direction calculated to preclude any possibility of union with O. This is understood by the psychotic patient, who does not resort to resistances but relies on being able to evoke the resistance-proliferating elements in his analyst; in other words, to stimulate the analyst's desires (notably for a successful outcome of the analysis), his memories, and his understanding, thereby intending that his analyst's state of mind will not be open to the experience of which he might otherwise be a witness.

This digression brings us back to the question of what is to be regarded as a fact. It appears to mean that the analysis should reinforce doubts of 'facts' which are part of 'memory'. The tendency to try to recall some supposed 'cause' of the crisis and to desire some different and more pleasing situation must be resisted. At best it can only recall some episode supposed to be the 'cause'. The 'recalled memory' saturates the psycho-analyst's pre-conceptions and obscures the issues at the one point where clarity of judgement and scope for its exercise are able to coincide – the current session.

To repeat: the capacity to forget, the ability to eschew desire and understanding, must be regarded as essential discipline for the psycho-analyst. Failure to practise this discipline will lead to a steady deterioration in the powers of observation whose maintenance is essential. The vigilant submission to such discipline will by degrees strengthen the analyst's mental powers just in proportion as lapses in this discipline will debilitate them. This view departs from commonly accepted practice and it may be as well, therefore, to consider the theoretical basis implicit in accepted practice.

The idea that patient A comes five times a week and has been doing so for months or years is based on a background of sense impressions and a view of the individual's continuity as an individual which is primitive and crude. It is the emergence of primitive number as a method of asserting 'constant conjunction', of asserting that the object is recurrent, that the 'breast' is something that reappears. We are not concerned with the patient's anatomy; a belief that no cellular changes take place in twenty-four hours is unwarranted on any but a crudely macroscopic view. The mental phenomena with which we are confronted cannot possibly have remained unaltered even if no analysis had been done. The mental phenomena should reveal invariance and it should be possible to observe the invariants embedded in these phenomena, but an invariant is a characteristic not of permanence but of transformation. It must be sought for in transformation. A psycho-analyst who remembers that A is the same person as A was yesterday indulges a column 2 element. Nor is there any reason for the analysand to believe that the analyst is the same person as the analyst of the previous day. Such belief is suspect as the sign of a collusive relationship intended to prevent emergence of an unknown, incoherent, formless void and an associated sense of persecution by the elements of an evolving O.

Desire, memory, understanding thus have the column 2 function of keeping F at bay and preventing the transformation in K from becoming transformation in O. Ostensibly they represent a compromise, for not only do they preclude F and transformations in O but they substitute transformations in K which give a similitude of transformation in O and make the pre-conception (D) in K serve as a saturation rather than as a means to a saturation. 'How I wish I had the chance to swim!' expresses the idea that a particular state of completion (wishing to swim) has been achieved and precludes the unsaturation that would be felt were the individual to *wish* to swim. Of all the hateful possibilities, growth and maturation are feared and detested most frequently. This hostility to the process of maturation becomes most marked when maturation seems to involve the subordination of the pleasure principle and the emergence of the reality principle. The change cannot be regarded as hated because it involves loss of pleasure, for the activity of the pleasure principle means activity of pain. Similarly, the continuation of pleasure when the dominance of the pleasure principle is in abeyance is not precluded by the dominance of the reality principle. But the change from pleasure principle to reality principle does mean abandonment of control over the proportion of pain to pleasure and leaves it to forces that are outside the personality. At-one-ment or unity with O is in prospect fearful. No experience challenging this preconception prevails because it is embodied in memory and desire, belongs to K, and does not transform into, though it may mark the inception of, O.

The central point appears to be the painful nature of change in the direction of maturation. It is probably idle to ask why it should be painful, why intensity of pain bears so little relationship to intensity of recognizable danger, and why pain is so feared. There is no doubt that mental pain in particular is feared in a way that would be appropriate if it corresponded directly with mental danger. The relationship of pain to danger is, however, obscure. In this it is not peculiar, for any relationship of one element of the personality with another seems difficult to determine. A science of relationships has yet to be established and one would look to find some discipline analogous to mathematics to represent the relationship of one element in the structure of the psychic personality with another. It is possible to argue that mathematical formulations can be fully appreciated because there is always some more concrete background to which they can be seen to relate, *even though that background may itself be only mathematical.* Something similar may be possible in the relationship of elements of the structure of personality. Envy is typical of other elements of the personality in that everyone would be prepared to admit its existence. Yet it does not smell; it is invisible, inaudible, intangible. It has no shape. It must have invariance, or it could not be so widely and surely recognized; and if it has invariants it must be invariant with regard to some kind of operation and therefore there must be an underlying group of such operations.

5 · Theories: Particular Instance or General Configuration

Controversy is the growing-point from which development springs but it must be a genuine confrontation and not an impotent beating of the air by opponents whose differences of view never meet. What follows is a contribution to bringing different psycho-analytic views together in agreement or disagreement.

Hearing psycho-analytic controversy I have felt that the same configuration was being described and that the apparent differences were more often accidental than intrinsic; different points of view are believed to be significant of membership of a group, not of a scientific experience. Yet everyone knows that what is important is not the supposed use of a particular theory but whether the theory has been understood properly and then whether the application has been sound.

It may be objected that to establish this would involve consideration of every individual analyst and of the circumstances of every individual interpretation. Even so, many difficulties could be obviated by more precise definition of the point of view (vertex). It is permissible for an observer to say that he has no evidence of infantile sexuality provided he also adds that he is an aeronautical engineer and does not take anything but a cursory view of children. What is *not* permissible is that he should say that he has no evidence of infantile sexuality without mentioning his vertex. I hope that there will be evolved a method of designating the vertex with brevity and precision. The following is a loose description, by way of a prelude to something more scientific.

To attain to the state of mind essential for the practice of psycho-analysis I avoid any exercise of memory; I make no notes. When I am tempted to remember the events of any particular session I resist the temptation. If I find myself wandering mentally into the domain of memory I desist. In this my practice is at variance with the view that notes should be kept or that psycho-analysts should find some method by which they can record their sessions mechanically or should train themselves to have a good memory. If I find that I am without any clue to what the patient is doing and am tempted to feel that the secret lies hidden in something I have forgotten, I resist any impulse to remember what happened or how I interpreted what happened on some previous occasion. If I find that some half-memory is beginning to obtrude I resist its recall no matter how pressing or desirable its recall may seem to be.

A similar procedure is followed with regard to desires: I avoid entertaining desires and attempt to dismiss them from my mind. (It is not enough to try to do this in the session because that is too late: the habit of desiring must not be allowed to grow.) For example, I think it a serious defect to allow oneself to desire the end of a session, or week, or term; it interferes with analytic work to permit desires for the patient's cure, or well-being, or future to enter the mind. Such desires erode the analyst's power to analyse and lead to progressive deterioration of his intuition. Introspection will show how widespread and frequent memories and desires are. They are constantly present in the mind and to follow the advice I am giving is a difficult discipline. There are exceptions, all of a simple and obvious kind.

Some matters can be easily recorded and need not burden the mind, as, for example, the times of sessions. It would be absurd if the analyst forgot to keep them and they are easily recorded on a timetable. The same may be true of age, members of the family, past illnesses, and other such facts as fancy might dictate. But these are to be recorded, together with addresses and telephone numbers, because they can then be forgotten and because they lend themselves to record. While it can be precisely stated that the patient is married and has four children it is not easily stated that his state of mind is that of a married man with four children because there is no such state of mind. Furthermore, such a 'memory', and the remembrancer that such a note would provide, would greatly obscure observation of the patient's state of mind suppose it were to be more nearly what one might expect of a bachelor.

Matters that can be recorded with the means at present at our disposal, including mental means, are sensuous experiences, and the transformations they undergo issue in formulations which have all, mathematical formulations included, a sensuous background. The central phenomena of psycho-analysis have no background in sense data. Even the signs that accompany anxiety, for example increased respiration, would be more appropriate to smelling a danger, if that danger had a scent and our olfactory powers were well developed, than to detecting an endo-psychic phenomenon. An apparatus that might be useful where a danger is sensible is useless or obstructive when the danger derives from a background that is mental and not sensible. Therefore, keep records for events whose background is sensible, such as the time at which a patient is to appear, but not for phenomena of central concern to the psycho-analyst, since their background is not sensible.

How, then, are we to 'observe' and 'record' the patient's state of mind? Since I wish to discuss this but do not know the answer, I shall say 'by F'.

Freud said that he had to 'blind myself artificially to focus all the light on one dark spot'.[1] This provides a useful formulation for describing the area I wish to cover by F. By rendering oneself 'artificially blind' through the exclusion of memory and desire, one achieves F; the piercing shaft of darkness can be directed on the dark features of the analytic situation. Through F one can 'see', 'hear', and 'feel' the mental phenomena of whose reality no practising psycho-

[1] In the letter referred to on p. 43 above.

analyst has any doubt though he cannot with any accuracy represent them by existing formulations.

The vertex I have thus far attempted to represent in this description may later be more accurately defined. Even as it is, I hope that my description will serve to make certain advantages clear. For example, it is easier for another psycho-analyst to appreciate my work if he knows the vertex and can thus anticipate what he thinks are its merits and defects. He does not have to engage in a barren argument about the theories I use (in a context of which he can know nothing) if he is given some idea of the state of mind in which I apply them.

It can be seen that with one vertex theories might be useful that are not useful with another; that if the vertex were altered other theories would be required to illuminate the phenomena discussed. Conversely, another psycho-analyst could understand that I might 'see' the oedipal situation in a context in which he might not.

The rules are relatively easy for a psycho-analyst to obey, and if they are obeyed dissimilar people with dissimilar patients may yet have a similar experience and so tend less often to mistake for general laws what are in fact only particular instances of old ones.

The experience to which I refer is the contact with the evolved aspects of O, the realization that I have variously described as ultimate reality, the thing-in-itself, or truth. Logically, in so far as logic affords a model for the approach I am making, the absence of memory and desire should free the analyst of those peculiarities that make him a creature of his circumstances and leave him with those functions that are invariant, the functions that make up the irreducible ultimate man. In fact this cannot be. Yet upon his ability to approximate to this will depend his ability to achieve the 'blindness' that is a prerequisite for 'seeing' the evolved elements of O.

Reciprocally, his freedom from being 'blinded' by the qualities (or his perception of them) that belong to the

58

domain of the senses should enable the analyst to 'see' those evolved aspects of O that are invariant in the analysand. The further the analysis progresses the more the psycho-analyst and the analysand achieve a state in which both contemplate the irreducible minimum that is the patient. (This irreducible minimum is incurable because what is seen is that without which the patient would not be the patient.)

Suppose the patient proliferates endless stories, coherent, plausible, and apparently true. After some analysis it becomes evident that something is wrong: the associations vary from accounts of episodes alleged to have happened and quite likely to have happened, to accounts that sound no less convincing but that reveal flaws. From internal evidence it is clear that the event could not have happened. But for incongruities, the tone of assurance of the narrative would have lulled all suspicion. If the narration is challenged the patient admits the fault and at once begins to proliferate further fabrications which invite the analyst either to withdraw his comments and acknowledge the truth of the patient's assertions or to say openly that he is lying.

It is not relevant to describe details of this case. By regarding the patient's statements as transformations and categorizing them by means of the grid, one can do something towards understanding what is taking place. I have advocated (in *Elements of psycho-analysis*) exercises of this kind but it must not be supposed that understanding of this nature is required. On the contrary, such 'understanding' can be seen to have as its background memory and desire and should therefore be avoided. The importance of the exercise is to facilitate the analyst's capacity for conjecture, not to intrude upon an analytic session. If the analysis is conducted as I advocate, the 'evolution of O' becomes manifest in the chains of fabrications such as I have described. It should be possible to observe a wide spectrum of categories of lies and what they represent. The flow of associations demands a high degree of inventiveness and speed (especially in sealing off any breach in the fabrications), and a measure of verbal facility that may give an impression of intelligence, especially if memory and desire distort judgement of the category. I am concerned here not with the diagnosis, prognosis, treatment, or cure, but with the O of psycho-analysis. From one vertex it might seem that the analysand was 'blinding' the analyst in that the analyst was flooded with illumination – so many facts that the 'obscure' point could not be 'seen'. Is this statement distinguishable from the state produced if the analyst is not successful in ridding himself of memory and desire? Only the psycho-analytic session can provide the answer. Extra-analytic activity stimulates doubt and curiosity in the analyst. Such a patient stimulates memory and desire by appearing to satisfy but without doing so; the analyst is tacitly invited to 'remember' all he is told.

A number of questions, of which the following are a few, are posed by this behaviour:

1. Are the patient's statements lies? Is 'lie' the most appropriate term to use? If not, what is the correct formulation?

2. Why does the patient transform in fabrications and what does he thus transform?

3. Does the fabrication differ from myth? It is often a plausible and coherent narrative, but it seems to declare itself to be category 3 when in fact it would appear to be C2. What, then, are the emotional experiences that are to be covered up and not allowed to emerge?

4. How do the patient's statements differ from other false statements? Respect for the truth appears to have low value compared with other vertices. What, then, is the vertex? – K? How does this compare with Plato's objections to the poet in society? With regard to other false statements it is usually supposed that there is either a mistaken idea that the lie is correct, or a belief that some reward attaches to being able to mislead. Some statements appear to be without reward to either party but perhaps there is a pleasure in creation even though creation can be achieved only by a lie. Is it a *folie à deux* – a

collaboration? Certainly with F it could be a sado-masochistic collusion to 'poison' or be 'poisoned'.

These questions can be answered only in analytic contact with the patient. The grid, or some improved version of it, facilitates mental gymnastics in preparation for it.

6 · The Mystic and the Group

It seems absurd that a psycho-analyst should be unable to assess the quality of his work. In attempting an assessment he has available popular repute (notoriously fickle and unreliable, and unsuited for use as a foundation for any judgement), anxiety, or a sense of satisfaction and well-being about a piece of work that appears to him to be well done. This last is probably as reliable a foundation as any, but is subject to doubt and misgiving. The only other person well placed to have an opinion is the analysand. His opinion is likewise a matter for scrutiny. The friendly or hostile feelings revealed converge towards a point where there should be a wise and compassionate, though critical, judgement. Instead there is an intuition, 'That is truth, accept it.' Such formulations are not regarded as scientifically adequate and one craves something better. The craving cannot be satisfied unless it is recognized that standpoints such as religion, art, science, as we understand them today, are as unsatisfactory as the formulations truth, beauty, god, or future life.

The formulation is the end-product of a transformation; all transformations are associated with a particular vertex. The psycho-analyst is faced at an early date in his own development and at an early stage in the development of psycho-analysis itself with problems that arise because no vertex at present recognized is adequate. It is as absurd to criticize a piece of psycho-analytic work on the ground that it is 'not scientific' as it is to criticize it because it is 'not religious' or 'not artistic'. It is not any of these things. Its failure to be so is a criticism; but its 'success' at being any of them would not remove the reproach. The critical formulation for which there is no substitute is that it is 'not psychoanalysis'.

62

It would seem that we are as far as ever from a positive result to the discussion; 'psycho-analysis' must be regarded as a term binding a constant conjunction. Years must pass before we understand what are conjoined and what the conjunction means. Can it be done in verbal terms? Are there any other terms?

It has been said in criticism of psycho-analysis that it cannot be regarded as a science because it cannot be mathematized. Available mathematics do not provide the psychoanalyst with appropriate formulations. The same is true of available verbalizations, but this has been obscured because ordinary conversation has served fairly well for the analysands who have come for analysis hitherto. This situation has been altered by the advent of so-called severe cases on the one hand, and by the needs of communication between psycho-analytic colleagues on the other. It is clear that a development is required that will help psycho-analysis in a manner analogous to that in which modern mathematics has helped the development of physics. In the meantime we are thrown back on existing verbal, mathematical, and artistic formulations and the exceptional individuals capable of employing them. Genius has been said to be akin to madness. It would be more true to say that psychotic mechanisms require a genius to manipulate them in a manner adequate to promote growth or life (which is synonymous with growth).

The group needs to preserve its coherence and identity; efforts to do so are manifested in conventions, laws, culture, and language. It also needs the exceptional individual and therefore needs to make provision for the exceptional individual. This might be simple if exceptional individuals declared themselves in unexceptionable terms and if the nature of their impact on the group, its laws and conventions, could be judged as life-giving or the reverse. The possibility of such discrimination is doubtful and, centuries after, it may still be debated whether an individual of this kind exerted a beneficial or deleterious effect. The same is true of ideas; furthermore, groups are hostile or friendly, favourable or unfriendly, to the development of the new person or idea.

The 'exceptional individual' may be variously described as a genius, a messiah, a mystic, and his following may be large or small. The negative group declares itself an enemy of promise in a manner that may not be discernible to ordinary individuals, but is apparently clear to the gifted individual who seeks an atmosphere more congenial to the exercise of his gifts. For convenience, I shall use the term 'mystic' to describe these exceptional individuals. I include scientists, and Newton is the outstanding example of such a man: his mystical and religious preoccupations have been dismissed as an aberration when they should be considered as the matrix from which his mathematical formulations evolved.

The mystic may declare himself as revolutionary or he may claim that his function is to fulfil the laws, conventions, and destiny of his group. It would be surprising if any true mystic were not regarded by the group as a mystical nihilist at some stage of his career and by a greater or less proportion of the group. It would be equally surprising if he were not in fact nihilistic to some group if for no other reason than that the nature of his contribution is certain to be destructive of the laws, conventions, culture, and therefore coherence, of a group within the group, if not of the whole group. In this it is evident that the character of the group, which I do not discuss, cannot be excluded from the facts of the evolution of a mystic in a group. The disruptive force of the mystical nihilist, or of the mystic whose impact on a particular group is of a disruptive or nihilist character, extends to and depends on the Language of Achievement, be it expressed in action, speech, writing, or aesthetic. Usually the spread of the disruptive force is limited by the vehicle of communication. The phenomena of destruction remain the same but reception of their message varies, often being restricted to relatively few.

Melanie Klein writes of symbol formation as if it were a particular function that could distintegrate or be disordered and give rise to deep disturbance in a personality; there are realizations that correspond to this theory, but I think the area of disturbance should be regarded as greater than her theory implies. For example, the psychotic patient does not always behave as if he is incapable of symbol formation. Indeed, he often talks or behaves as if he is convinced that certain actions, which to me are innocent of any symbolic significance, are obviously symbolic. They mean, apparently obviously, some message which is of personal and particular concern to him. This 'meaning' is quite different from the meaning one assumes to lie behind a constant conjunction that is public and not private to one individual. The former is, and appears to belong to, a private communication made by God (or Devil or Fate); when the psychotic symbol is met with in practice its significance seems to be less that it symbolizes something, more that it indicates that the patient is in private rapport with a deity or demon. The symbol, as it is usually understood, represents a conjunction which is recognized by a group to be constant; as encountered in psychosis it represents a conjunction between a patient and his deity which the patient feels to be constant.

The 'symbol' can be an attempt of the personality to use its experience to formulate a theory, which may then be used when the appropriate realization presents itself, or an attempt to use an external event, e.g. a meeting with an acquaintance, to yield an interpretation *as if it were* a symbol. Thus an adverse circumstance can be used as a 'symbol' (not 'sign') of God's wrath, or past experiences can be represented by symbols whose genetic base is in their *sensuous* background. The emotional experience is thus made manageable by being symbolized, whether it is in origin felt to be a response to a painful external stimulus, or whether the external experience is felt to be the confirmation of a painful internal psychic experience.

The inescapable bestiality of the human animal is the

quality from which our cherished and admired characteristics spring. 'Man is a political animal' means that he has the mental counterpart of the physical characteristics of a herd animal. As psycho-analysts, we are concerned with the mental counterpart of such physical characteristics as can be discerned in the individual when in semi-isolation from his group, but closely involved in a situation likely to stimulate his 'pair' characteristics. Birth, dependence, pairing, and warfare – these are the basic situations to which the basic emotional drives correspond.

This summary of the human condition adds nothing new to what is already familiar, in greater detail, to every psychoanalyst. The summary is intended as a reminder that the analytic situation itself, and then the psycho-analytic occupation or task itself, are bound to stimulate primitive and basic feeling in analyst and analysand. Therefore, if the technique I propose for ensuring vivid appreciation of the emotional facts is as sound as I think it, these fundamental characteristics, love, hate, dread, are sharpened to a point where the participating pair may feel them to be almost unbearable: it is the price that has to be paid for the transformation of an activity that is *about* psycho-analysis into an activity that *is* psycho-analysis. The activity that is psychoanalysis evokes desires to know how the group is reacting to the pair relationship; this desire often masquerades as a wish for validation, popular repute, or approval.

We thus return to the original problem (p. 6f. above) and the impulse to repudiate the approach I have adumbrated. The more reminiscence is indulged, the farther one is removed from a form of anxiety: one's historical identity is asserted, one was such and such and had certain recognized and remembered associates; one has done as well as, or less well than, so and so. It is doubtful whether these 'historical' reminiscences would be corroborated by any of the characters who figure in one's own story, but they serve to deny the painfulness of the actual predicament that is the source of embarrassment. It is difficult, short of hallucination, to do anything about the present predicament: reminiscence becomes a C2 category orgy to keep out the painful insights that follow on denial of sensuous experience.

There is one form of denial of sensuous experience that has been a commonplace since Freud pointed out that analysis must be conducted in an atmosphere of deprivation.[1] It has not been recognized that to achieve this it is not enough to hope that analysis of the analyst and denial of the patient's wishes will serve. Anyone who considers it possible to achieve a suitable frame of mind by a few minutes of psychological tidying up before starting work cannot have grasped the nature of the discipline necessary to be an analyst or the nature of the insights that become available to the analysed analyst if he brings 'artificial blindness' to bear on his dark spots. It may well be that analysts who attempt the approach advocated in Chapter 4 on 'Memory and Desire' will find that the intuitions achieved by it cause them to feel the need for further analysis. It is possible that the test of sensuous deprivation involved in eschewing memory and desire will bring to light a need for analysis that exists because the analytic experience has not been sufficient, or it may be that it indicates an *additional* demand that would not have occurred had the analyst remained content with the 'atmosphere of deprivation' as it has been understood hitherto. The point is of moment because, if the abandonment of memory and desire brings a need for increased stamina, analysts may have to accept that advances in insight have to be matched by further analysis. Such a contingency imposes revision of training and maintenance of capacity for a psycho-analytic career.

Though it is easy to envisage the need for further analysis, it is not certain that the further analysis must be similar to analysis as experienced and understood when we undergo our first analysis. The importance of the unconscious must not blind us to the fact that in addition to our unconscious memories and desires, dealt with psycho-analytically, there

[1] Discussed in detail in a paper by Dr Samuel Futterman of Los Angeles.

is a problem to solve in the handling of our conscious memories and desires. What kind of 'psycho-analysis' is required for the conscious?

The psychotic *is* conscious of what we feel requires analysis; to approach this problem it will be necessary to discuss memory and desire relative to loss of contact with reality. It has been supposed that the psychotic severs links with reality as a step to a sexual life in phantasy, but it is equally intended to establish freedom from sexual and allied stimulation. He appears to achieve a result resembling the neurotic patient's contact with the unconscious as it is known in classical analysis. The psychotic seems to have the same relationship and attitude to what he has *not* been able to repress, and what therefore remains conscious, that other patients have to the unconscious. The neurotic patient is concerned to show that neurotic elements in his behaviour are rational and does his best to rationalize them. The psychotic can 'see' that any action has a symbolic meaning and that the conjunction of the elements is not fortuitous but has a meaning which is clear *to him*. This is possible provided he has severed all links with anything that shows the conjunction to be fortuitous and devoid of meaning, that is, in my terminology, unsaturated – a D category element. The premature saturation involved in this has the paradoxical effect that all acts are symbolic and yet the patient is incapable of symbol formation in the way open to the normal personality who can allow his elements to remain unsaturated. Contact with reality is unwelcome because it tends not only to show that an element is unsaturated but also to saturate the element in ways that are painful to the personality. As all his 'symbols' have an obvious meaning they can hardly be regarded as symbols at all and nothing is left that can fulfil the function that symbols fill for the non-psychotic personality.

How does this differ from the state produced by the elimination of memory and desire?

First, I am advocating only a partial severance with

reality. Second, it is a deliberate, conscious act of discipline. Third, it has a purpose that would appear to differ from the purpose of the psychotic manoeuvre. He wishes to destroy contact; I wish to establish it. Furthermore, he is primarily concerned with destruction of sensuous contact and its concomitant saturation whereas I am anxious to diminish sensuous contact to bring psychic reality into focus. The psychotic fears and hates that result; it is an extension of reality.

The domain of personality is so extensive that it cannot be investigated with thoroughness. The power of psychoanalysis demonstrates to any practising psycho-analyst that adjectives like 'complete' or 'full' have no place in qualifying 'analysis'. The more nearly thorough the investigation, the clearer it becomes that however prolonged a psycho-analysis may be it represents only the start of an investigation. It stimulates growth of the domain it investigates. This difficulty I mean to exploit in this way: if it is true that the proportion of the known to the unknown is so small at the *end* of analysis, it must be even smaller *during* analysis. Therefore to spend time on what has been discovered is to concentrate on an irrelevance. What matters is the unknown and on this the psycho-analyst must focus his attention. Therefore 'memory' is a dwelling on the unimportant to the exclusion of the important. Similarly, 'desire' is an intrusion into the analyst's state of mind which covers up, disguises, and blinds him to, the point at issue: that aspect of O that is currently presenting the unknown and unknowable though it is manifested to the two people present in its evolved character. This is the 'dark spot' that must be illuminated by 'blindness'. Memory and desire are 'illuminations' that destroy the value of the analyst's capacity for observation as a leakage of light into a camera might destroy the value of the film being exposed.

To consider objections to the elimination of memory: it may seem impossible to have a link with a patient without remembering who he or she is; but such recognition does not depend on memory, nor does psycho-analysis. It depends on a background of an experience the peculiarity of which I shall indicate by a series of approximations. We are familiar with the experience of *remembering* a dream; this must be contrasted with dreams that float into the mind unbidden and unsought and float away again as mysteriously. The emotional tone of this experience is not peculiar to the dream: thoughts also come unbidden, sharply, distinctly, with what appears to be unforgettable clarity, and then disappear leaving no trace by which they can be recaptured. I wish to reserve the term 'memory' for experience related to conscious attempts at recall. These are expressions of a fear that some element, 'uncertainties, mysteries, doubts',[1] will obtrude.

Dream-like memory is the memory of psychic reality and is the stuff of analysis. That which is related to a background of sensuous experience is not suitable to the phenomena of mental life which are shapeless, untouchable, invisible, odourless, tasteless. These psychically real (in the sense of belonging to psychic reality) elements are what the analyst has to work with.

It may appear that this contradicts the psycho-analytic theory of dreams unless it is remembered that the dream is the *evolution* of O where O has evolved sufficiently to be represented by sensuous experience. The sensuous elements of a psychotic dream do not represent anything. They *are* a sensuous experience.[2]

Anyone who has made careful notes of what he considers to be the facts of a session must be familiar with the experience in which such notes will, on occasion, seem to be drained of all reality: they might be notes of dreams made to ensure that he will not forget them on waking. To me it suggests that the experience of the session relates to material akin to the dream, not in the sense that dreams might be part

---

[1] John Keats, 'Letter to George and Thomas Keats', 21 December 1817.
[2] The use of the sensuous experience to represent a psychic reality differentiates the neurotic dream and its symbolic quality from the psychotic dream.

of the preoccupation of the session but that the dream and the psycho-analyst's working material both share dream-like quality.

The *reality* of the psychic experience – the O in the human personality – is such that the more the analyst is in contact, the more real will be that part of it that he has been able to interpret. It will be clear to him that he is formulating only one aspect of a multi-dimensional experience. What will dwell in his mind will be the multi-dimensional experience. Once he has interpreted it the facet that he has interpreted ceases to be of moment. The psycho-analyst reads his notes with a sense of an emotional experience powerfully present in his mind, but it is of an experience of the as-yet unknown. It is against this powerful sense that he reads the note of an event which ceased to be of importance when it was formulated. The attempt to remember or record destroys the capacity for, and interrupts the exercise of, observation of the psycho-analytically significant events.

Conversely, the sacrifice of memory and desire is conducive to the growth of dream-like 'memory' which is a part of the experience of psycho-analytical reality. The transformation of the emotional experience into mental growth of analyst and analysand contributes to the difficulty of both to 'remember' what took place; in so far as the experience contributes to growth it ceases to be recognizable; if it does not become assimilated it adds to those elements that are remembered and forgotten. Desire obstructs the transformation from knowing and understanding to being, $K \rightarrow O$.

7 · Container and Contained

An advantage of believing that observations are the foundation of scientific method is that the conditions in which they are made can be stated and then produced. The simplicity of this has its appeal for the psycho-analyst: an analytic situation is presumed to exist and interpretations of the observations made in that situation are then reported. It is possible to believe that the analysis has a location in time and space: for example, the hours arranged for the sessions and the four walls of the consulting-room; that at such times and in such a place the analyst can make observations which he cannot do if the domain has not these limitations, or if 'psycho-analytic observations' do not conform to the conventional view of an observation. If I pictorialize the statement 'the conventional view of an observation' to be a container, like a sphere, and the 'psycho-analytic observation' as something that cannot be contained within it, I have a model that will do very well not only for the 'conventional view', to represent my feelings about a 'psycho-analytic situation', but also for the 'psycho-analysis' that it cannot contain. It will also serve as a model for my feelings about certain patients: I cannot observe Mr X because he will not remain 'inside' the analytic situation or even 'within' Mr X himself.

I have found theories of acting-out enlightening, but not enlightening enough; none of the theories known to me 'contains' the 'facts' by which I seek to be enlightened. My 'facts' gird against the framework of definition and theory which I seek to erect around them. The patient who is acting out cannot be 'contained' within existing formulations.

This is a characteristic of the mental domain: it cannot be contained within the framework of psycho-analytic theory. Is this a sign of defective theory, or a sign that psycho-

72

analysts do not understand that psycho-analysis cannot be contained permanently within the definitions they use? It would be a valid observation to say that psycho-analysis cannot 'contain' the mental domain because it is not a 'container' but a 'probe'; the formulation that I have tried to further by using the symbols ♀ and ♂ minimizes this difficulty by leaving ♀ and ♂ as unknowns whose value is to be determined.

I would pursue this train of thought further by discussing something more practical and particular. It is a matter where action[1] seems to be called for, namely, the institutionalization of psycho-analysis comprising publication, selection, training, and qualification.

In recent years there has grown up the use of the term Establishment; it seems to refer to that body of persons in the State who may be expected usually to exercise power and responsibility by virtue of their social position, wealth, and intellectual and emotional endowment. (This list is not an order of priority of attainments.) I propose to borrow this term to denote everything from the penumbra of associations generally evoked, to the predominating and ruling characteristics of an individual, and the characteristics of a ruling caste in a group (such as a psycho-analytical institute, or a nation or group of nations). Because of my choice of subject it will usually be used for talking about the ruling 'caste' in psycho-analytical institutes.

The Establishment has to find and provide a substitute for genius. One of its more controversial activities is to promulgate rules (known in religious activities as dogmas, in scientific groups as 'laws', e.g. of nature or perspective) for the benefit of those who are not by nature fitted to have direct experience of *being* psycho-analytic (or religious, or scientific, or artistic) so that they may, as it were by proxy, have and impart knowledge of psycho-analysis. Group members will not through incapacity be denied a sense of participation

---

[1] I shall include psycho-analysis itself in the category of 'action' for reasons given under the heading of Language of Achievement in Chapter 13.

in an experience from which they would otherwise feel for ever excluded. At the same time these rules (or dogmas) must be such that they attract rather than repel, help rather than hinder, the membership of genius, which is essential to the group's continued existence and vitality. A Freud can discover and establish psycho-analysis, but it must be maintained by a continued supply of 'genius'. This cannot be ordered; but if it comes the Establishment must be able to stand the shock. Failing genius, and clearly it may not materialize for a very long period, the group must have its rules and a structure to preserve them. Thus an environment exists ready, as Nietzsche said of the nation, to fulfil its proper function, namely, to produce a genius. Similarly, it may be said of the individual that he should be ready to produce a 'flash of genius'. Let us therefore consider this phenomenon.

The term 'genius' does not carry the associations I want, so I propose to use the term 'mystic', leaving it to be supposed that the mystic has characteristics usually associated with genius and that the person represented by the term 'genius' or 'mystic' may with equal propriety be described by the term 'messiah'.

The mystic is both creative and destructive. I make a distinction between two extremes that coexist in the same person. The extreme formulations represent two types: the 'creative' mystic, who formally claims to conform to or even fulfil the conventions of the Establishment that governs his group; and the mystic nihilist, who appears to destroy his own creations. I mean the terms to be used only when there is outstanding creativeness or destructiveness, and the terms 'mystic', 'genius', 'messiah' could be interchangeable.

The problem posed by the relationship between the mystic and the institution has an emotional pattern that repeats itself in history and in a variety of forms. The pattern may appear in the relationship of a new phenomenon to the formulation that has to represent it. It appears in the relation-

74

ship of widely dissimilar groups to their mystics; it reveals itself in the history of the Christian heresies, the heliocentric theories, the relationship of the rabbinical directorate of the Kabbalah to revolutionary mystics such as Isaac Luria, the political reformer, and the Establishment.

My object is to show that certain elements in the development of psycho-analysis are not new or peculiar to analysis, but have in fact a history that suggests that they transcend barriers of race, time, and discipline, and are inherent in the relationship of the mystic to the group. The Establishment cannot be dispensed with (though this may appear to be approximately achieved in Sufism and in the theory of Marxism) because the institutionalized group, the Work group (see Bion, 1961), is as essential to the development of the individual, including the mystic, as he is to it. Homeric psychology indicates a stage of mental development in which the distinction between man and god is ill defined; in the individual psyche, little distinction between ego and super-ego is recognized. The Work group, under the religious vertex, must differentiate between man and god. Institution-alized religion must make man conscious of this gulf in himself and in the counterparts of himself in the group of which he is a member.

The institutionalization of psycho-analysis requires a psycho-analytic group which has 'Establishment' as one of its functions. It is itself a replica, in the external world, of an object in which the desired separation has been effected. But its function is then to effect this separation in the personalities of its members. It is thus both a model of a state that is desired and an institution whose function it is to make the individual aware of the gap between himself (his idealized, super-egoized self) and himself (his unregenerate, un-psycho-analysed self).

One result of separation is no direct access of the individual to the god with whom he used formerly to be on familiar terms. But the god has undergone a change as a part of the process of discrimination. The god with whom he was

75

familiar was finite; the god from whom he is now separated is transcendent and infinite.

To restate the above in terms appropriate to a background of human experience: Freud and his associates mix on terms of equality such as exist between any human colleagues in a common venture. Freud, merely by being a person of outstanding stature, stimulates the tensions and emotional drives appropriate to a primitive group and stimulates them still further by his work. The primitive stages of the analytic group contribute to the obtrusion of tensions and emotional drives appropriate to the primitive group, as Freud observed through his study of the individual. I doubt that he appreciated the force of the messianic hopes aroused. The primitive stage makes way for the stage of discrimination described in the religious group: a distinction is made, otherwise there will not be recognition of the real distinction that exists between a mystic (in my sense) and ordinary human beings.

This distinction cannot be achieved adequately by saying that it is inseparable from idealization. Idealization in the group is a reality-based activity which is essential for the growth of discrimination in the individual. The individual himself must be able to distinguish between himself as an ordinary person and his view that he is omniscient and omnipotent. It is a step towards recognition of a distinction between the group as it really is and its idealization as an embodiment of the omnipotence of the individuals who compose it. Sometimes the separation fails and the group is not only seen to be ideally omnipotent and omniscient but believed to be so in actuality. The individual's realization of a gulf between his view of himself as omnipotent and his view of himself as an ordinary human being must be achieved as the result of a task of the group itself as well as in individual analysis. Otherwise there is a danger that a state of mind is transferred (by projective identification) to the group and *acted out* there – not altered. Some details of this situation must be described.

76

In the first stage there is no real confrontation between the god and the man because there is really no such distinction. In the second stage the infinite and transcendent god is confronted by the finite man. When the function of the group is to *establish* the separation there is no question of reunion. In the third stage the individual, or at least a particular individual – the mystic – needs to reassert a direct experience of god of which he has been, and is, deprived by the institutionalized group. Before I turn to this it is necessary to glance at some peculiarities of the group that has been institutionalized and of life in it.

The individuals show signs of their divine origin (just as the gods of the previous stage show signs of human origin). The individuals may be regarded as being incarnations of the deity; each individual retains an inalienable element which is a part of the deity himself that resides in the individual. He can be regarded as constantly attempting to achieve union with the deity, or he can be regarded as divine in a somewhat low-grade way. This last shows signs of being related genetically to the stage where no real distinction exists between god-like human beings on the one hand and very human gods on the other. Finally, the individual strives for reunion with the god from whom he feels consciously separated. This is reflected in the actualities of the human relationship and contributes to the hatred of the group for a state in which individuals cannot have direct access, or even a sense of direct access, to the great man (as they might once have had to Freud). Individuals cannot reconcile themselves to a discrimination that means conscious separation of themselves from a belief in their Freud-like qualities and recognition that Freud, a genius (mystic), no longer exists. Another Freud cannot be created no matter how essential he may be.

The group and mystic are essential to each other; it is therefore important to consider how or why the group can destroy the mystic on whom its future depends and how or why the mystic may destroy the group. I shall indicate the nature of the questions at issue since it is vital that the problem should be seen to exist. It is inherent both in the nature of man as a political animal and in the nature of psycho-analysis as the explosive force.

The relationship between group and mystic may belong to one of three categories. It may be commensal, symbiotic, or parasitic. The same categorization may be applied to the relationship of one group with another. I shall not trouble with the commensal relationship: the two sides coexist and the existence of each can be seen to be harmless to the other. In the symbiotic relationship there is a confrontation and the result is growth-producing though that growth may not be discerned without some difficulty. In the parasitic relationship the product of the association is something that destroys both parties to the association. The realization that approximates most closely to my formulation is the group–individual setting dominated by envy. Envy begets envy, and this self-perpetuating emotion finally destroys host and parasite alike. The envy cannot be satisfactorily ascribed to one or other party; in fact it is a function of the relationship.

In a symbiotic relationship the group is capable of hostility and benevolence and the mystic contribution is subject to close scrutiny. From this scrutiny the group grows in stature and the mystic likewise. In the parasitic association even friendliness is deadly. An easily seen example of this is the group's promotion of the individual to a position in the Establishment where his energies are deflected from his creative–destructive role and absorbed in administrative functions. He epitaph might be 'He was loaded with honours and sank without a trace'. Eissler (1965), without mentioning the general principle involved, shows the dangers of the invitation to group or individual to become respectable, to be medically qualified, to be a university department, to be a therapeutic group, to be anything in short, but *not* explosive. The reciprocal attitude in the mystic is that the group should thrive or disintegrate but must *not* be indifferent. The attitudes are not conscious and deliberate; they are essential. Without them the group is not a group nor the 'mystic' a

78

mystic. An analytic parallel is the psycho-analytic interpretation which is death to the existing state of mind, the
state of mind that is being interpreted. Worse than being
right or wrong is the failure of an interpretation to be significant, though to be significant is not enough; it merely
ensures that it exists. It must also be true. The parasitic
group can be primarily concerned to destroy the mystic, or
mystic (messianic) ideas, but if it fails to do so it must
'establish' his or their truth.

Eissler discusses 'applied' psycho-analysis. I suspect that
applied psycho-analysis, even if 'applied' to curing people, is
a method of bringing psycho-analysis under control and
rendering it harmless to the Establishment. I have expressed
this in another context and in a different approach by a rule
that the analyst should not permit himself to harbour
desires, even the desire to cure, since to do so is inimical to
psycho-analytical development. Development itself is not an
object that can be 'desired'. The painful nature of the
dilemma is essential.

The recurrent configuration is of an explosive force with a
restraining framework. For example, the mystic in conflict
with the Establishment; the new idea constrained within a
formulation not intended to express it; the art form out-
moded by new forces requiring representation.

It is essential that the language should be preserved. To
this end, rules are produced under which words and definitions are to be used. The *Oxford dictionary*, linguistic philosophy, mathematical logic, are tributes to the work that is
incessantly proceeding for this purpose. On this work
ordinary men and women with ordinary ability depend to do
work that otherwise would be done only by exceptional
people. Thanks to Faraday and other scientists ordinary
people can illuminate a room by the touch of a switch;
thanks to Freud and his co-workers ordinary people hope by
psycho-analysis to be able to illuminate the mind. The fact
that the world's work has to be done by ordinary people
makes this work of scientification (or vulgarization, or

simplification, or communication, or all together) impera-
tive. There are not enough mystics and those that there are
must not be wasted.

The more successfully the word and its use can be
'established', the more its precision becomes an obstructive
rigidity; the more imprecise it is, the more it is a stumbling-
block to comprehension. The new idea 'explodes' the formulation designed to express it. Sometimes the emotion is
powerful but the idea weak. If the formulation survives it can
be repeated. If it can be repeated under severe conditions it
becomes stronger until it communicates meaning without
distintegration. Conversely, the formulation may destroy its
content. In his play *Major Barbara*, George Bernard Shaw
describes the apotheosis of the dictum 'No man is good
enough to be another man's master' as a method of rendering
the emotional content ineffectual.

It may be that the distinction between creative and
nihilistic mystic is no more than a temporary expedient
depending on the need to express one view of the mystic
rather than the other. The most powerful emotional explosion known so far, spreading to many cultures and over
many centuries, has been that produced by the formulations
of Jesus. The effects are still felt and present grave problems
of containment even now, though some measure of control
has been established. Jesus at first expressly disavowed any
aim other than fulfilment of the laws of his group. The
rabbinical directorate failed to solve the problem of containment, a failure associated with disastrous consequences
for the Jewish group. The disaster attributed to Christian
teachings did not terminate at any finite point, as for example at the crucifixion; after Alaric had sacked Rome four
hundred years later St Augustine felt the reproaches against
the Christians to be sufficiently serious to require refutation
in his 'City of God'.

The problems of mystical revelation that centre on having, or claiming to have, a direct relationship with the deity
remain. The need for the Establishment to do what the rab-

binical directorate had failed to do soon became evident. Complaints by the disciples that miracles were being done by unauthorized or, as we might say, 'lay', people, suggest awareness that we expect to find associated with an Establishment. That, and evidence of a need to establish a structured hierarchy ('who shall sit at the right hand'), is too slender to be more than a starting-point for conjecture. Something must have contributed to the efflorescence of structure, hierarchy, and institution. The institution is evidence of the need for the function that the rabbinical directorate had failed to provide. Although in many respects the Church was more successful, the long history of heresy (see Knox, 1950) shows that the structure required to contain the teaching of Jesus was, and still is, subjected to a great strain. It has not, however, been without its successes, and even today complaints can be heard, which are really a tribute to the success of the institutionalizing process, of the lack of enthusiasm, drive, and 'spirituality' of the Church.

Though we may contrast the success of the Church favourably with the failure of the rabbinical directorate, the force of the mystical revelation has not yet spent itself. There are signs that the Oedipus myth, and the elements that in the Christian religion touch on paternity and sonship, both have a configuration suggesting an underlying group of which these elements are representative. I have used the sign O to denote this 'ultimate reality'. Any formulation felt to approximate to illumination of O is certain to produce an institutionalizing reaction. The institution may flourish at the expense of the mystic or idea, or it may be so feeble that it fails to contain the mystical revelation.

A formulation may approximate to 'illumination' of O. Many mystics express their experience of direct access to the deity in terms of light, but light is not the only model used. Jewish mystics in particular find the voice a telling representation of the experience. St Paul found light *and* voice necessary to represent the experience. It is significant that psycho-analysts seeking direct access to an aspect of O,

81

though it is not only to that part of O that informs god-like characteristics, conduct their affairs through language. To be confined to one medium of communication only is too restrictive even if it has the flexibility and capacity for development of language. Psycho-analytical observation certainly cannot afford to be confined to perception of what is verbalized only: what of more primitive uses of the tongue?

The suspension of memory and desire promotes exercise of aspects of the psyche that have no background of sensuous experiences. Paradoxically, the release of these aspects of the psyche enables them to reveal elements such as the non-verbal muscular movements of the tongue, as in stammer. The dominance of sensuous experience promotes expressions such as 'seeing' or 'hearing'; the falseness introduced by such formulation contributes to those differences that seem so significant but are in fact unimportant. Intuitive power cannot develop because it is hindered by such obtrusions of 'sense'. The institutionalizing of words, religions, psycho-analysis, – all are special instances of institutionalizing memory so that it may 'contain' the mystic revelation and its creative and destructive force. The function of the group is to produce a genius; the function of the Establishment is to take up and absorb the consequences so that the group is not destroyed.

8 · Vertices: Evolution

Some psycho-analytic tensions appear in a simpler, less disguised form if we use as a model the impact of the thought of Jesus on the Jewish group and on later religious institutions. The stress on miracles of healing represented an urge to 'medicalize' the institution intended to serve the teaching of Jesus. Healing retains its dominance in Christian Science, Lourdes, faith-healing. An example in the early Christian group of a problem of institutionalizing is the query put to Jesus by the disciples who wanted to have a ruling on recognition of those who cast out devils in Jesus' name. His attitude appears to have been against rigid qualification for membership of the group – 'those that are not against me are for me'. Although this reply cannot now be interpreted with sureness and may have been referable to the favourable (for Christianity) effect of turpitude in the opponents of Christianity, it shows the recurrent configuration of the problem of selection (lay versus professional, or outgroup versus ingroup). These conjectures illustrate the configuration to which I want to draw attention.

Psycho-analysis cannot escape ideas of cure, treatment, illness, in psycho-analysts and patients alike. Eissler warns against a structure that is too rigid and too limited to permit development. At the opposite extreme the Sufis have no rigid institution yet have endured; their solution would open the way for an 'expanding universe' of psycho-analysis but it would not be long before members of the psycho-analytic movement could not understand each other.

The importance of unconscious motivation has tended to screen the importance of conscious motivation. An analyst or a particular group of analysts may stress a medical view possessing, in my terms, a common vertex; an observer of

83

the group would expect to find that its vertex is recognized by certain invariants such as ideas of disease, treatment, prognosis, pathology, and cure. The unconscious counterparts of such a vertex will have been laid bare in the psychoanalysis of the individuals, but this should not blind us to the conscious aspects of this vertex.

Suppose a group in whom the need or desire to make money is obtrusive. The unconscious counterpart of this will likewise have been laid bare in the analysis of the individuals. The greater the need or the 'desire', the easier it would be to detect a particular application of psycho-analytic theory (what Eissler calls 'applied' psycho-analysis as opposed to 'anthropic').

Other groups may display similarly obtrusive vertices: a wish for power, influence, propaganda, education, research, or poverty. It is evident that, in our present stage of development, if we achieve 'psycho-analytic' psycho-analysis, the vertex of the group will make a difference to the findings of the group. So far, analysts have seemed to act on the assumption that motives should be analysed and may, therefore, be safely left without further consideration. This view ignores the varieties of development opened up by the analytic experience.

The oedipal situation, or its even more primitive roots, would have a different configuration according to whether the vertex of the group was psycho-analytic, religious, financial, legal, or some other. This itself increases the variety of experiences opened up within the limits of even rigid psychoanalysis. The messianic expectation, formulated and institutionalized in the Christian religion, may represent the evolved aspect of an element which is represented also at its evolved stage by the Oedipus myth.

Similarities in the configurations suggest a common origin and common disorders associated with the problem of containing the mystic and institutionalizing his work. The emotional impact of ♀♂ will be proportionately greater the more closely it is related to the forces represented by the messianic hope, the Oedipus myth, the Babel myth, and the Eden myth; the greater the emotional impulse the greater the problem. These myths are evolved states of O and *represent* the evolution of O. They represent the state of mind achieved by the human being at his intersection with the evolving O.

Where Eissler speaks of applied psycho-analysis I shall speak of psycho-analysis conducted from a particular vertex. If an analyst or group of analysts regards the making of money as an essential part of psycho-analytic practice, that is to say that they regard it as an essential part of practice which is an equally essential part of cure, then I think that the vertex should be described as money-making and the discoveries that are made in such analysis will bear the stamp of the financial vertex.

If the vertex is religious I should expect the discoveries to bear the stamp of that vertex. In time, the configurations associated with the various vertices would evolve to a point where they could be formulated. I should then expect the rigidity conferred by the formulation to be resisted by the fluidity of the O represented by the formulation. Just as there is at present an unbridged gap between the animate and the inanimate, which makes the transformation of the inanimate into the animate impossible, so there is a gap between the formulation of the configuration and the underlying realization approximating to it. The configuration that represents the relationship between the mystic and the institution can be recognized in, and be the representation of, the relationship between the emotional experience and the representative formulation (words, music, painting, etc.) designed to contain it. The same configuration can be seen in the relationship between the Dionysian emotional experience and the Apollonian representation. Direct access to the O of the mystic and the O of the Dionysian orgy is both contained and restrained by the religious dogmas substituted for them in the minds of 'ordinary' people.

Most analysts have felt at some time that the 'universe of discussion' in psycho-analysis is expanding so fast that we no longer maintain what a soldier calls 'lateral communication'. To take one instance about which I am able to have an opinion: the gap between what some regard as analysis and what I, as a Kleinian, regard as analysis is very wide and widening. This is attributed to differences in theory. I do not believe that what separates scientists is their difference in theory. I have not always felt 'separated' from someone who differs from me in the theories he holds; that does not seem to me to afford a standard of measurement by which the gap can be measured. Conversely, I have felt very far separated from some who, apparently, hold the same theories. Therefore, if the 'gap' is to be 'measured' it will have to be in some domain other than that of theory. The differences in theory are symptoms of differences in vertex and not a measure of the differences.

9 · Ultimate Reality

So far this book has been concerned with the formulation of a theory, the few 'facts' mentioned being illustrative models intended to give body to what might otherwise be an exercise in the manipulation of abstractions. It leads up to the formulation of a theory which has as its realization a background of psycho-analytic practice. The theory formulates a recurrent pattern of emotional experience of wide distribution. It does not replace any existing psycho-analytical theory, but is intended to display relationships which have not been remarked.

However thorough an analysis is, the person undergoing it will be only partially revealed; at any point in the analysis the proportion of what is known to what is unknown is small. Therefore the dominant feature of a session is the unknown personality and not what the analysand or analyst thinks he knows.

All psycho-analytic progress exposes a need for further investigation. There is a 'thing-in-itself', which can never be known; by contrast, the religious mystic claims direct access to the deity with whom he aspires to be at one. Since this experience is often expressed in terms that I find it useful to borrow, I shall do so, but with a difference that brings them closer to my purpose. The penumbra of associations is intended to help those who look for my meaning.

In any object, material or immaterial, resides the unknowable ultimate reality, the 'thing-in-itself'. Objects have emanations or emergent qualities or evolving characteristics that impinge upon the human personality as phenomena. Of these qualities the personality may be consciously or unconsciously aware; they differ from the ultimate reality.

'Ultimate reality' is a term with a penumbra of associations, which makes it psychologically helpful, but this fact

87

makes it unsuitable to represent something that by definition is unknowable. The same objection applies to the term 'godhead'. Meister Eckhart expresses his sense that the godhead evolves to a point where it becomes apprehensible by man as the Trinity.

By contrast the godhead is formless and infinite. Milton expresses a similar idea in the description of the world of waters dark and deep which has been 'won from the void and formless infinite', though here the emphasis is less on the evolution characteristic of the godhead and more on the capacity of the apprehending object to apprehend.

The religious approach postulates an emanation of the deity and an incarnation of the deity. Both formulations are needed to represent states of mind in which there is an interaction between states of an object that is sometimes whole, sometimes split into fragments dispersed within a multiplicity of objects. For the analyst, the doctrine of the incarnation yields the rewarding model so I shall concentrate on it first.

The psycho-analyst witnesses the behaviour of a being who is usually, but not always, lying on a couch and talking. The analyst may take in the scene as a whole or any part of it. 'Whole' or 'part' is an aspect of an ultimate reality that has evolved until it intersects the personality of the observer (see Chapter 3 above).

The scientific approach, associated with a background of sense impressions, for example the presence of the psycho-analyst and his patient in the same room, may be regarded as having a base. In so far as it is associated with the ultimate reality of the personality, O, it is baseless. This does not mean that the psycho-analytic method is unscientific, but that the term 'science', as it has been commonly used hitherto to describe an attitude to objects of sense, is not adequate to represent an approach to those realities with which 'psychoanalytical science' has to deal. Nor is it adequate to represent that aspect of the human personality that is concerned with the unknown and ultimately unknowable – with O.

The criticism applies to every vertex, be it musical, religious, aesthetic, political; all are inadequate when related to O because, with the possible exception of the religion of the mystic, these and similar vertices are not adapted to the sensually baseless. The realities with which psycho-analysis deals, for example fear, panic, love, anxiety, passion, have no sensuous background, though there is a sensuous background (respiratory rate, pain, touch, etc.) that is often identified with them and then treated, supposedly scientifically. What is required is not a base for psycho-analysis and its theories but a science that is not restricted by its genesis in knowledge and sensuous background. It must be a science of at-one-ment. It must have a mathematics of at-one-ment, not identification. There can be no geometry of 'similar', 'identical', 'equal'; only of analogy.

The Platonic theory of Forms and the Christian dogma of the Incarnation imply absolute essence which I wish to postulate as a universal quality of phenomena such as 'panic', 'anxiety', 'fear', 'love'. In brief, I use O to represent this central feature of every situation that the psycho-analyst has to meet. With this he must be at one; with the *evolution* of this he must identify so that he can formulate it in an interpretation. Certain states of mind obstruct this and of them I shall say more later.

An aspect of O that evolves is signified by number. Participating in the evolution can be the object, which may multiply or decrease, and the observer, who feels that the object multiplies or decreases. Ignoring the object so as to discuss only the observer one may say that he *feels* that the object increases or decreases. The constant conjunction signified by number excites curiosity to know which, what, when, why, or how. 'The need to know' (whether the change ($\pm$) is in the objects observed or in the 'feeling') may be activated. The 'number' is assumed to relate to an aspect of the object observed, but it may with equal propriety be regarded as relating to the feeling. I shall be discussing mostly the 'number' as being the name of the feeling, but to avoid confusion I shall distinguish between, say, R3 (external reality) and $\psi 3$ (psychic reality), the latter being the sign for a feeling of 'threeness' which may or may not be contemporaneous with 'threeness' as an aspect of the observed object.

When I speak of 'number', in the context of feelings, the term has too many associations that I do not require. I shall therefore use (ξ) to denote the name of a 'mathematical object'[1] which I am using as the name of a 'feeling'.

The following illustrations, taken from religion, politics, conversational intercourse, and so on, may act as an introduction to 'psychical' mathematics:

'The majority of people . . .'
'Thousands (millions) all over the world . . .'
'The Trinity'
'Four or five people . . .'
'For weeks (months, years) they waited for . . .'

In these examples, numbers, used to represent a feeling in the observer, may be categorized in accordance with the principles of the grid as intended to evoke curiosity (category 4) or as a barrier against statements that might evoke a psychological disturbance (category 2).

These 'numbers' have been transformed from ψ (ξ) to R (ξ), so that they represent realizations which approximate to them. These realizations can become extremely complex. Thus Euclidean geometry has been regarded as a representation to which space, as ordinary people know it, is the approximate realization. Euclidean geometry then becomes the background realization that approximates to axiomatic algebra, which represents *it*.

Axiomatic algebra appears to be entirely independent of its background and can be developed accordingly; on the theory developed here, although it may start by representing feelings that provide the background, axiomatic algebra, the example I have taken, becomes entirely independent of that

[1] Borrowed from Frege (1950).

background of feelings. The H formulations (grid category) begin to lack 'body'. What does it mean that these formulations lose 'body', cease to represent a 'feeling'? The number 'three' or 'ten' can easily represent a 'feeling' that there are three or ten objects present. The names three and ten do not seem to represent constant conjunctions in the way that 'cat' does. 'Cat' has a sensuous background; so has $R(\xi)$; but $\psi(\xi)$ has not unless we reverse a process of transformation through Euclidean geometry back to ordinary space. Non-sensuous phenomena form the totality of what is commonly regarded as mental or spiritual experience. $\psi(\xi)$, which represents non-sensuous realizations, seems to be relatively easily adapted for manipulations to represent *sensuous* realizations, but not for manipulations to represent non-sensuous realizations. If 'three' represents a non-sensuous realization of 'threeness', why can it not, in combination with 'ten', 'five', etc., be made to represent anxiety or love or hate?

Certain problems can be handled by mathematics, others by economics, others by religion. It should be possible to transfer a problem, that fails to yield to the discipline to which it appears to belong, to a discipline that can handle it. If Euclidean geometry cannot handle multi-dimensional problems they can be transferred to algebraic geometry which can handle them. In this way certain problems can be transferred within their own discipline so that their solution can be attempted. The mathematics evolved by the manipulation of 'numbers' has so far proved very successful in matching the formulation with the realization it represents. But the numbers representing feelings have not evolved so that they can handle the realizations of the domain from which they appear to have sprung.

Before we consider the transference of problems from one discipline to another, or of the procedures proper to one discipline to procedures proper to another discipline, we shall examine the peculiarities of catastrophic change.

10 · Visual Images and
Invariants

From the material discussed it should now be possible to detect a pattern that remains unaltered in apparently widely differing contexts. It would be useful to isolate and formulate the invariants of that pattern so that it could be communicated.

Freud's formulations do just that. Thinking, developed through psycho-analysis, has led to discoveries that were not made by Freud, but that reveal configurations resembling those in discoveries he *did* make. Can his formulations be replaced by others that reveal as nearly as possible *all* the configurations that are similar and not merely those instances that his formulations were intended to illuminate?

If his Oedipus theory is used in conjunction with the Eden myth, the Babel myth, and a version of messianic expectation, it can continue to illuminate the mind's workings as it does now and to display elements of an underlying configuration that widen significantly the area illuminated. The deity's hostility to curiosity remarked by Milton's Satan (Book IV, *Paradise Lost*) can be matched in Babel by the attack on speech (the infliction of confusion of tongues); in Oedipus by Tiresias and his warning; in the messianic story by the attack on the son by the father. The same pattern is reflected in the self-inflicted punishments of the Sphinx and Oedipus. Each version emphasizes a different facet; together they suggest a common configuration. The attempt to differentiate emotional elements is curiously unsuccessful. Thus 'omnipotent good', 'evil', 'pursuit of knowledge through curiosity', 'impending disaster', 'arrogance', and so on, each attempt seems to weaken the impact that the elements have

92

when they are part of the narrative as a whole; they undergo a transformation similar to that undergone by the dream upon being consciously recalled, or by a work of art when it is replaced by a reproduction. The transformation depends on a change of vertex. The vertex of the myth-maker is not mine as I attempt this reformulation; the vertex of the dreamer is not that of the dreamer awake; the vertex of the artist is not that of the interpreter of the work of art. Similarly, the vertex of the psycho-analyst, and changes of vertex corresponding to moment-to-moment changes in a session, effect the transformations made manifest in associations and interpretations.

First, there must be a difference of vertex to make correlation possible. It must ultimately take place in the individual. (For the moment I assume that correlation is a necessary part of confrontation and that confrontation is a necessary part of analysis.) Schizophrenic defences are mobilized against confrontation; violence makes confrontation impossible because both sides of a confrontation are annihilated.

Second, the vertex must not be too distant or too near, otherwise correlation becomes impossible. How is 'distance' measured between the vertex of the analysand and the vertex of the analyst? If the analyst wants to make a living and the analysand wants to be 'cured', how is the 'distance' between these vertices to be 'measured'? A man and a woman can have such different outlooks that their temperaments are described as incompatible; or views so similar that they cannot stimulate each other. Is there any sense in which their views can be so 'far apart' that the distance can be 'measured', that a phrase used metaphorically can be treated so that the metaphorical sense is replaced by a literal sense?

Under this vertex the views of patient and analyst are separated; the 'gap' separating them is bridged by something that I call linear or planar, or a line or film. Very different is the gap that is bridged by a relationship between container and contained. The following will serve as a model for a theoretical formulation of this kind of link: a man speaking

93

of an emotional experience in which he was closely involved began to stammer badly as the memory became increasingly vivid to him. The aspects of the model that are significant are these: the man was trying to contain his experience in a form of words; he was trying to contain himself, as one sometimes says of someone about to lose control of himself; he was trying to 'contain' his emotions within a form of words, as one might speak of a general attempting to 'contain' enemy forces within a given zone.

The words that should have represented the meaning the man wanted to express were fragmented by the emotional forces to which he wished to give only verbal expression; the verbal formulation could not 'contain' his emotions, which broke through and dispersed it as enemy forces might break through the forces that strove to contain them.

The stammerer, in his attempt to avoid the contingency I have described, resorted to modes of expression so boring that they failed to express the meaning he wished to convey; he was thus no nearer to his goal. His verbal formulation could be described as like to the military forces that are worn by the attrition to which they are subjected by the contained forces. The meaning he was striving to express was denuded of meaning. His attempt to use his tongue for verbal expression failed to 'contain' his wish to use his tongue for masturbatory movement in his mouth.

Sometimes the stammerer could be reduced to silence. This situation can be represented by a visual image of a man who talked so much that any meaning he wished to express was drowned by his flood of words.

I hope that I have conveyed my meaning to the reader by virtue of the verbal transformations of visual images that I have used. However, the communication is not satisfactory. The visual images are too concrete to be suitable for expressing the relationship of the mystic to the group. They are too evocative of a penumbra of associations which they already carry. In short, the situation is similar to that of the stammerer whose words, or lack of them, contain rather than

94

communicate his meaning. Alternatively, the meaning is too powerful for the verbal formulation; the expression is lost in an 'explosion' in which the verbal formulation is destroyed. To consider the essentials: the communication is about a relationship between meaning and its expression, between emotion and its expression. But I am aware that it is not a relationship between any things; it is a pattern of relationships in the way that mathematicians speak of mathematics as expressing relationships. I have in the past used the symbols ♀ and ♂ to express a relationship between container and contained; for the present I shall continue to do so.

The theory is that an object is placed into a container in such a way that either the container or the contained object is destroyed. In pictorial terms the container is represented by a mouth or vagina, the contained by breast or penis. The relationship between these objects, which I shall represent by the male and female signs ♂ and ♀, may be commensal, symbiotic, or parasitic.

By 'commensal' I mean a relationship in which two objects share a third to the advantage of all three. By 'symbiotic' I understand a relationship in which one depends on another to mutual advantage. By 'parasitic' I mean to represent a relationship in which one depends on another to produce a third, which is destructive of all three.

Take another simple visual model: a man wishing to communicate his annoyance is so overwhelmed by emotion that he stammers and becomes incoherent. The invariants under the theory I wish to formulate are the forms of speech that the man uses to convey his meaning; these I regard as being intended to 'contain' what he has to say and therefore to correspond to the sign ♀. The annoyance he strives to communicate I regard as being what should be contained in his speech, and therefore it is appropriately represented by ♂. If the man remained coherent, this could correspond to an overwhelming of the content by the container: his speech would in this case be so restrained that it could not express his feelings. But suppose he expressed himself 'perfectly':

one could then imagine that his emotions had served to develop his ability for well-chosen speech and that his capacity for speech had helped his emotional development. This contrasts with development leading to incoherence. Such a failure is the outcome of a 'parasitic' relationship between the contained (or rather, *not* contained) material and the speech devised to contain it: 'container' and 'contained' have produced a third 'object' – incoherence – which makes expression and the means of expression impossible. In so far as the imaginary episode led to a development of powers of expression and of the personality that strove to express itself, the relationship could be described as symbiotic. 'Commensal' is illustrated by supposing that the episode occurred in an age and society (as in Elizabethan England) in which language had reached a point of development where the ordinary man was inspired to speak it well: that which was to be expressed and the vehicle for its expression profited from the culture to which they belonged.

11 · Lies and the Thinker

The distinction between truth and lie constantly confronts the psycho-analyst who has to apply in a rough and ready practical way ideas that have been the centre of discussion over the centuries. The rough and ready application may be too crude to do the work required of it. The psycho-analyst seeks ideas sufficiently accurate and robust to survive the emotional storms they should illuminate.

To the problems of understanding I have said that the psycho-analyst can bring something that is unknown to the philosopher of science because the psycho-analyst has experience of the dynamics of *misunderstanding*; the psycho-analyst is concerned *practically* with a problem that the philosopher approaches *theoretically*. Investigations of understanding and misunderstanding impinge on problems associated with truth and untruth. The reality of the problem becomes apparent when the psycho-analyst must ask himself, can a liar be psycho-analysed?

The problem can be formulated in grid terms without moral overtones. Category 2 (reserved for formulations known by the initiator to be false but maintained as a barrier against statements that lead to a psychological upheaval) would seem provisionally to offer a home to the lie. Such a categorization supposes that an experience has been permitted to continue to a point where the patient thinks he knows his formulation to be untrue, but is it true that he maintains it because it would be disturbing to his development not to do so? The lie could be uttered because in the view of the liar it would be profitable to him or injurious to another: is it correct in such a case to say it would be true, and if true significant, that inability to profit himself or injure another would lead to his having a psychological upheaval?

97

As I think it would be true, I must indicate why and in what way it is reasonable to categorize the lie in 2. First I am concerned with patients who come for analysis and not with those who do not. To such a patient it is clear that he risks exposure of the lie. He must either have great confidence in his capacity (or lack of it in the analyst) or feel some dissatisfaction with the lie. These are random conjectures, however, and beg the question at issue, which must be answered in the course of an analysis the very practicability of which is under debate. The extreme case would seem to offer the best chance of being able to observe the essential characteristics, or, as I prefer to call them, the invariants, of the liar. Present considerations make it unlikely that the psychoanalyst would treat such a case by choice. The supposition that he was going to cure such a patient would lead him to hesitate about accepting him. Therefore the probability is that the lying is so well concealed that he stumbles into such a collaboration unwittingly. This makes it possible that the same may be true of the patient; so at the outset one must be prepared to find that the supposition that the patient thinks he risks exposure, or minds it if he does, is not in fact the case.

The need for a category for statements known by the patient to be untrue arises when, for example, a patient, who has been shown in the course of analysis that there are a number of explanations of the fact that he is late, continues to repeat apologies. The analyst is challenged to accept them, at the risk of showing himself unmindful of the truth, or to reject them and assume the role of being the patient's conscience. A statement may be made not to mislead but to fill the function of evocation. Thus a lying report may be evocative or provocative, accusatory or defensive, to name only a few of the more obvious uses. In such a case category 2 is not the correct category because the statement is intended to lead to emotional upheaval. In short, the lying statement is not category 2 but category 6. Its nature must be indicated by some usage such as minus L $(-L)$ or minus K $(-K)$.

The term 'lie' thus has limited value for use in the course

of psycho-analysis. It focuses attention on something that is not invariant; on the other hand, $-L$ or $-K$, together with the appropriate grid category, leaves it open to saturation by appropriate 'meanings' should realizations that approximate present themselves to the psycho-analyst and analysand.

If we suppose now that the emotional upheaval against which the lie is mobilized is identical with catastrophic change it becomes easier to understand why investigation uncovers an ambiguous position which is capable of arousing strong feelings. These feelings relate to an outraged moral system; their strength derives from risk of change in the psyche. As the episode that I describe occurs frequently and can be resolved only in a way that seems to set the pattern for the resolution of subsequent recurrences, it is necessary to dwell on certain features which have an importance that may escape notice.

The patient can be seen to make a decision between the lie and the truth. The frequency with which this 'decision' is automatically made in favour of the statement known to be untrue will determine the nature of the case. I focus attention on the position that now arises for the analyst.

By definition and by the tradition of all scientific discipline, the psycho-analytic movement is committed to the truth as the central aim. If the patient constantly formulates $-L$ and $-K$ statements, he and the analyst are, in theory at least, in conflict. In practice, however, the situation does not present itself so simply. The patient, especially if intelligent and sophisticated, offers every inducement to bring the analyst to interpretations that leave the defence intact and, ultimately, to acceptance of the lie as a working principle of superior efficacy. In the last resort he will make consistent progress towards a 'cure' which will be flattering to analyst and patient alike. The alternative he offers is bleak: progressive deterioration, loss of mutual esteem both private and public, hostility, and, in extreme cases, threats of legal action. Against this the analyst has to balance a hope of retaining his integrity.

Some forms of lying appear to be closely related to experiencing desire. Long stories, with every appearance of truth, are spun out extempore as if the virtuosity of the exercise gave pleasure. One would expect such fabrications to be idealizations, and some are, but the liar's state of mind is not ordinary and the divergence from the usual is screened by the plausibility of his lies. They are usually C category formulations and may present more difficulty to an analyst whose mind is built on sensuous experience than to one who is used to discounting memory. As the problems of the psycho-analysis of the liar differ so much from those of the psycho-analysis of one whose outlook is scientific, it is worth considering shortly what is meant by the scientific approach. In ordinary speech it is taken to mean an assumption that the truth is of overriding importance and that reason should be harnessed to its elucidation. As a preliminary to attempting a more sophisticated formulation the opposite view may be stated in terms of fable, thus:

The liars showed courage and resolution in their opposition to the scientists who with their pernicious doctrines bid fair to strip every shred of self-deception from their dupes leaving them without any of the natural protection necessary for the preservation of their mental health against the impact of truth. Some, knowing full well the risks that they ran, nevertheless laid down their lives in affirmations of lies so that the weak and doubtful would be convinced by the ardour of their conviction of the truth of even the most preposterous statements. It is not too much to say that the human race owes its salvation to that small band of gifted liars who were prepared even in the face of indubitable facts to maintain the truth of their falsehoods. Even death was denied and the most ingenious arguments were educed to support obviously ridiculous statements that the dead lived on in bliss. These martyrs to untruth were often of humble origin whose very names have perished. But for them and the witness borne by their obvious sincerity the sanity of the race must have perished under the load placed on it. By laying down their lives they carry the morals of the world on their shoulders. Their lives and the lives of their followers were devoted to the elaboration of systems of great intricacy and beauty in which the logical structure was preserved by the exercise of a powerful intellect and faultless reasoning. By contrast the feeble processes by which the scientists again and again attempted to support their hypotheses made it easy for the liars to show the hollowness of the pretensions of the upstarts and thus to delay, if not to prevent, the spread of doctrines whose effect could only have been to induce a sense of helplessness and unimportance in the liars and their beneficiaries.

It is not necessary to elaborate this phantasy further; this sample should indicate the vertex I wish to establish, but in so far as it does so it throws up difficulties. It is easy to imagine that there are such things as facts independent of the mind. A belief that led a man to throw himself off a cliff in confidence that his capacity to fly would preserve him from injury would contribute to his injury because the reality of his belief, the O of his belief, is, from the vertex of survival, of less consequence than the O of throwing himself from a cliff. But O, without such a vertex, is an absolute, inhering in ('incarnate' in) everything and unknowable by man. The belief that he would fly off uninjured can be compared with the belief that he would break his neck. Depending on the vertex, the two beliefs can be regarded as valuable and precedence accorded to one of them. But to what scale of values is the value of the belief related? Ruskin defined 'valuable' as life-giving. This may do in that the oedipal theory and primal scene afford a link (as does the theorem of Pythagoras, by the use of Cartesian co-ordinates, for the conversion of geometry to algebraic formulation) between life instincts and death instincts and that which is valuable or life-giving and its opposite.

If value is to be the criterion, difficulty arises because there is no *absolute* value: the individual does not necessarily believe it is better to create than to destroy; a suicidal patient may seem to embrace the opposite view.

The determination of the system of beliefs, the vertices, aims, complaints, and 'cures', is often mistaken by the patient for an attempt to establish a correct system. The investigation of category 2 is to see in what respect its pains compare with those of other systems and in what way the relationships differ. Such insights laid at the disposal of the patient seem to give him the opportunity to correct errors. The contemplation of various systems enables the analyst to reconsider and correct his own system. Category 2 involves conflict with impressions of reality; sometimes these may not matter but beyond a certain point the conflict between the need to know and the need to deny becomes acute and may usher in attacks on linking to stop stimulation which leads to conflict. But this presupposes an aim on the part of the liar, and therefore a pattern that can be detected. This is not the case with some liars. Hence it is not possible to rely on picking up a symptom, such as a wish to please the analyst, that will betray the pattern.

For satisfaction, the liar needs an audience; this makes him vulnerable, since his audience must set a value on his fabrications. It is therefore necessary that the analyst-victim should attach importance to the patient's statements as formulations of a truth. It must be possible to observe incoherent elements and to detect a pattern that brings together the disparate elements, showing a coherence and a meaning that they had not without it. So far, this description does not differ from that of the transformation from the paranoid–schizoid to the depressive position. It is superior to a narrative formulation which betrays the lying element of the story only by the weakness of the causative links. The Ps $\leftrightarrow$ D reaction reveals a whole situation which seems to belong to a reality that pre-exists the individual who has discovered it. The lying discovery lacks the spontaneous bleakness of the genuine Ps $\leftrightarrow$ D. The lie requires a thinker to think. The truth, or true thought, does not require a thinker – he is not logically necessary.

Provisionally, we may consider that the difference between a true thought and a lie consists in the fact that a thinker is logically necessary for the lie but not for the true thought. Nobody need think the true thought: it awaits the advent of the thinker who achieves significance through the true thought. The lie and its thinker are inseparable. The thinker is of no consequence to the truth, but the truth is logically necessary to the thinker. His significance depends on whether or not he will entertain the thought, but the thought remains unaltered.

In contrast, the lie gains existence by virtue of the epistemologically prior existence of the liar. The only thoughts to which a thinker is absolutely essential are lies. Descartes's tacit assumption that thoughts presuppose a thinker is valid only for the lie.

The paranoid–schizoid state may then be seen as peculiar to the thinker who is in a state of persecution by thoughts that belong to a non-human system, the O domain. The O domain may be said to be, *vis-à-vis* the thinker, in a state of evolution. This evolving system intersects with the personality of the individual thinker. The impact of the evolving O domain on the domain of the thinker is signalized by persecutory feelings of the paranoid–schizoid position. Whether the thoughts are entertained or not is of significance to the thinker but not to the truth. If entertained, they are conducive to mental health; if not, they initiate disturbance. The lie depends on the thinker and gains significance through him. It is the link between host and parasite in the parasitic relationship.

The relationship between the lie, the thought, the thinker, and the group is complex. The thinker may express the truth in a lying group; the group may not want its ideas disturbed and will be dominated by category 2 mechanisms and formulations. The relationship between such a group and such a thinker will be one of envy and hate. If the thinker is expressing lies, the relationship of the thinker to his lies will be parasitic, and lies and thinker will destroy each other. If the lie is of the 'sun rises at dawn' type, the relationship between lie and thinker is commensal – such a thought *requires* a thinker and the thinker is essential. But the relationship, at least in our present age, is commensal. The thought that the world will endure may be a lie but it may be essential to keep at bay ideas that the world is on the verge of coming to an end. Such a relationship between lie and thinker is symbiotic.

The link between one mind and another that leads to destruction of both is the lie. The term 'link' gives an inadequate idea of the realization it is intended to represent. The lie is not restricted, as the word 'lie' would ordinarily imply, to the domain of thought, but has its counterpart in the domain of being; it is possible to be a lie and being so precludes at-one-ment in O.

In psycho-analysis the liar is a significant fact and gains significance from the lying nature of what he says. The parasitic relationship between liar and environment, corresponding to the parasitic relationship between the thinker and the lie, denudes the environment of significance. The analyst who accepts such lies is acting as host; if he does not he contributes to the feelings of persecution by 'being' an unthought thought, a thought without a thinker. The thought to which a thinker is not necessary is also a thought that the thinker would not regard as likely to contribute to *his* significance. On the contrary, once he has expressed a truth the thinker is redundant.

To summarize, I formulate two definitions:

1. True thought requires neither formulation nor thinker.
2. The lie is a thought to which a formulation and a thinker are essential.

The lie is peculiar to a relationship between the host mind and the parasitic mind and destroys both. The thinker can harbour thoughts if he does not need thoughts to contribute to his significance and can tolerate thoughts that do not do so. If essential to the thought, the thinker conflicts with other thinkers who feel themselves to be essential to the thought. The envy, jealousy, and possessiveness aroused are the mental counterparts of toxic elements in physical parasitism.

They contribute to the destructive nature of the culture that develops from the development of the lie. The need for each individual to claim his contribution to the thought as unique and essential differentiates the emotional climate from that in which the inevitability of the thought and the unimportance of the individual who harbours it do not gratify the narcissism of the individual and therefore lack emotional appeal. Work that corroborates the discovery of others has a lack of appeal. Even if it requires a thinker it does not require a *particular* thinker and in this resembles truths – thoughts that require no thinker.

Since the analyst's concern is with the evolved elements of O and their formulation, formulations can be judged by considering how necessary his existence is to the thoughts he expresses. The more his interpretations can be judged as showing how necessary *his* knowledge, *his* experience, *his* character are to the thought as formulated, the more reason there is to suppose that the interpretation is psychoanalytically worthless, that is, alien to the domain O.

12 · Container and Contained Transformed

In this chapter I repeat the configuration in formulations that appear to be descriptions of events in psycho-analysis or history but have not the status of historical narrative. They are C category elements, images derived from a background of experience or reported experience, reassembled for my purpose.

Description 1: The signs ♂ and ♀ I call the contained and the container. The use of the male and female symbols is deliberate but must not be taken to mean that other than sexual implications are excluded. These signs designate a relationship between ♀ and ♂. The link may be commensal, symbiotic, or parasitic.

Description 2: A word contains a meaning; conversely, a meaning can contain a word – which may or may not be discovered. The relationship is established by the nature of the link. A constant conjunction of elements in a psycho-analysis can be 'bound' by the attribution to it of a word, a theory, or other formulation. The word by which it is bound can have such a powerful pre-existing penumbra of associations that it squeezes the meaning out of the constant conjunction it is supposed to mark. Conversely, the constant conjunction can destroy the word, theory, or other formulation that the formulation is intended to 'contain'. For example, a man is attempting to express such powerful feelings that his capacity for verbal expression disintegrates into a stammer or a meaningless, incoherent babble of words.

Description 3: The container (♀) extracts so much from the contained (♂) that the contained is left without substance. A

106

psycho-analysis is so long continued that the patient can get no further meaning from it. A converse example would be the continuation until the patient had no more patience, tolerance, fortitude, or money left. The container can squeeze everything 'out of' the contained; or the 'pressure' may be exerted by the contained so that the container disintegrates. An illustration would be the word used as a metaphor until the background is lost and the word loses its meaning.[1]

Description 4: The marriage *in* which the sexual relationship ♀♂ plays such a part that there is *no room* for any of the other activities in which the married couple might engage. Conversely, the other (i.e. 'other than sexual') activities play such a part that there is *no room* for sexual fulfilment. (The metaphors used in this description exemplify the outside–inside, container–contained, ♀♂ pattern.)

♀ or ♂ may represent memory. The container ♀ is filled with 'memories' derived from sensuous experience. The sensuous background is dominant and 'memories' with such a background are tenacious. The ♀ memory is saturated accordingly. The analyst who comes to a session with an active memory is therefore in no position to make 'observations' of unknown mental phenomena because these are not sensuously apprehended. There is something that has often been called 'remembering' and that is essential to psycho-analytic work; this must be sharply distinguished from what I have been calling memory. I want to make a distinction between (1) remembering a dream or having a memory of a dream and (2) the experience of the dream which seems to cohere as if it were a whole, at one moment absent, at the next present. This experience, which I consider to be essential to evolution of the emotional reality of the session, is often called a memory, but it is to be distinguished from the experience of remembering. In memory, time is of the essence. Time has often been regarded as being of the

---

[1] See H. W. Fowler's *Dictionary of modern English usage,* 2nd edition, 'Metaphor' 2D.

essence of psycho-analysis; in the growth process it has no part. Mental evolution or growth is catastrophic and timeless. I shall use 'memory' with its ordinary conversational meaning; it represents something that is out of place in the psycho-analyst's conduct of a psycho-analysis. A patient's close relatives are burdened with memories which make them unreliable judges of the patient's personality and unfit to be the patient's analyst.

So far, I have examined the configuration as it appears in the limits of words themselves; its appearance in more complex formulation indicates the degree of its persistence. The psycho-analytic situation provides and evokes examples of the configuration; it pervades difficulties which analysand and analyst find in communication. There are emotional experiences to be conveyed or represented, some of great intensity. Therefore, we find instances of the configuration in the subject-matter and in the psycho-analytic procedure designed to deal with it.

Description 5: The patient will be at a loss to convey his meaning, or the meaning he wishes to convey will be too intense for him to express properly, or the formulation will be so rigid that he feels that the meaning conveyed is devoid of any interest or vitality. Similarly, the interpretations given by the analyst, ♂, will meet with the apparently co-operative response of being repeated for confirmation, which deprives ♂ of meaning either by compression or by denudation. Failure to observe or demonstrate the point may produce an outwardly progressive but factually sterile analysis. The clue lies in the observation of the fluctuations which make the analyst at one moment ♀ and the analysand ♂, and at the next reverse the roles. When this pattern is observed the links (commensal, symbiotic, or parasitic) within the pattern must also be observed.

The more familiar the analyst becomes with the configuration ♀ and ♂, and with events in the session that approximate to these two representations, the better. The

108

essential experience is not the reading of this volume but the matching of the real event in the psycho-analysis that approximates to these formulations. The frequent references made to events that occur 'in analysis' or 'in the past' or 'inside' or 'outside' should aid recognition of the realizations to which these signs relate. The recognition of the category of link that is operating may be more difficult unless a lead-in can be obtained by considering the kind of event that takes the place of ♀ or ♂. Thus an extremely greedy patient may want to obtain as much as he can from his analysis while giving as little as possible; we should expect this to show itself by frequent events in which the container was denuding the contained object, and vice versa. The patient might show that he made enormous demands on his family but resented doing anything for it. Many patients might show behaviour of this kind on relatively rare occasions, but some might show it in many activities and in striking degree as, for example, by habitual incoherence while demanding great precision of interpretation from the analyst. This kind of patient cannot well be described in terms of narrative recording actual events, first, because any such formulation is suspect for reasons I have given in discussing memory, and, second, because it is impossible to predict what form his greed will take. Therefore the psycho-analyst who may have such a patient, or a patient showing such patterns of behaviour relatively rarely, or anything between these extremes, needs formulations of theory that enable him to have as wide a spectrum of observation as possible so that these configurations do not pass unnoticed. If these formulations are too abstract they lack body. Accordingly I give them body by using C category descriptions, but these are liable to produce so great a penumbra of associations that the formulations become saturated and narrow the psychoanalyst's perspicacity.

Descriptions 1–5 could include claustrophobia, agoraphobia, and acting-out as illustrations of the configuration.

Acting-out, as it is ordinarily understood, takes place 'in' the analysis and the analysis is then itself a part of acting-out. The claustrophobic-agoraphobic patient identifies himself with an object which is inside or outside a container. An ability to see the configuration reveals relationships within the patient's personality that otherwise would remain unknown. When a patient can be said to be acting out the analysis is 'in' a situation of which the boundaries are unknown. If the behaviour characterized as 'acting-out' is brought to the analysis it can be accompanied by claustrophobic symptoms in the patient. The coherence of these symptoms may not be detected if the underlying configuration is not realized. As this last point touches on group behaviour I shall make my next description a formulation in terms of history. The description will appear to be complex because I intend to broaden the scope of the configuration but its complexity will be less if it is borne in mind that the description has the same fundamental configuration even if at first sight it appears that this is not so. It may help if I explain that new ideas may appear to be presented in this description; their novelty or otherwise is a function of the reader's personality and must not be supposed to inhere in the communication.

Description 6: This section is mostly recapitulation and expansion of the model of mystic and group. Some mystics attract notice but others do not because the conditions are not propitious. The same is true of ideas. The idea which I consider to be the counterpart of the mystic or genius I call the 'messianic idea'. The idea that is messianic may be confused with the person; he may believe he is the messiah. The person I call 'the mystic'; the idea I call the 'messianic idea'. The terms 'mystic' and 'genius' are interchangeable. Mystics appear in any religion, science, time, or place. Such persons 'contain' the 'messianic idea' or the 'messianic idea' may 'contain' the person who is sought to incarnate, represent, or manifest the messiah in a manner analogous to the meaning that is felt to 'contain' the word that is to represent it.

The society in which the mystic appears has been described by Nietzsche as a body whose function it is to produce a genius. It is also the function of the society to make the mystic or messianic idea available to the members of the group. This is effected by laws (in society), dogma (in religion), rules or laws (in mathematics or science). The governing body of the society I call the Establishment; the counterpart in the domain of thought would be the pre-existing disposition or pre-conception.

The mystic makes direct contact with, or is 'at one' with, God. This capacity is not attributed to the ordinary member of the group. The Establishment must pronounce dogmatically, make laws or rules, so that the advantages of the mystic's communion with God or ultimate truth or reality may be shared at one remove by the ordinary members. This the Establishment may fail to do through lack of discrimination, leading to the furtherance of false views, or through rigid adherence to an existing framework, so that a parasitic link is set up between mystic and group, ♂ and ♀. The life is then squeezed out of the mystic or messianic idea or the society is disrupted.

Description 7: The conflict between the mystic and his group is exhibited in its most exaggerated, and therefore most easily studied, form in the account of Jesus and his relationship with the group. He himself claimed, in a manner typical of many mystics, that his teachings were in conformity with the existing Establishment: 'Think not that I am come to destroy the law or the prophets: I am not come to destroy but to fulfil' (Matthew 5 : 17, A.V.). This claim is often associated with an awareness of the disruptive force that is being brought to bear upon the group from within. The mystic does not always claim to conform to the group. He may appear in the guise of a destroyer from within or without. He does not claim peaceable intentions or methods. A

111

distinction is sometimes made between the nihilistic mystic, who disrupts the community, and the creative mystic, who denies violent methods particularly against his own group. I wish to stress the disruptive quality of the mystic, whether he claims to be disruptive or not, for it is this disruptive quality that is associated with the group's hostility to the mystic, and vice versa. It is, furthermore, the quality that I wish to emphasize in this description.

The reaction of the Establishment is to prevent the disruption, and this it does by incorporating the mystic within itself. This is expressed in the biblical illustration by the temptation in the wilderness where the rewards of conformity are clearly stated. Conformity can be renunciation of the messianic idea or acceptance of the role of the messiah. Alternatively, the mystic can be destroyed and an attempt made to ensure the same fate for his ideas.

The functions of containment – I use the word with its military implication of one force containing another – had to be assumed by the split factions of the group, one ostensibly against and the other for Jesus. Gradually a fresh group was formed and a fresh Establishment to contain the mystic or rather the messianic idea. The Jewish group learned to handle the mystic with consequences that were less disastrous for itself. The Christian group, though finding a different solution of the problem, achieved a similarly satisfactory result. Neither system was free from recurrences of the problem. One Christian Establishment restored the disrupted structure and ensured its continuity by taking over the festivals of paganism and thus mollifying the hostility that might otherwise have followed the loss of holidays and feasts that were beloved and valued. The theme could be stated as bigger and brighter paganism, with gods refurbished and rejuvenated as saints and devils. (Milton expresses this very clearly in his representation of Pandemonium in Books I and III of *Paradise Lost*.)

The problems of the Christian Establishment developed in the lifetime of Jesus. They were: delineation of the borders of the group, selection and training, and stabilization of the hierarchy.

To take the last point first. In the account in Mark's Gospel (10:35–45), the problem was clearly posed by James and John with their request for status. In his reply Jesus seems to suggest a kind of initiation or test, but the alacrity with which the two accept the conditions makes it hard to know what the initiation was, though it is clear that Jesus regarded its performance as beyond them. He also adumbrates a change in the function of the Establishment as it existed among the Gentiles of that time. The proposal put forward by James and John seems to be for status, and status appears to be a substitute for qualification. Their desires were to be satisfied as it were *ex officio*. The reply given by James seems to indicate that the 'position' achieved *ex officio* was an alternative preferred by the pair to undergoing the experience of the mystic himself. In this respect the rejected solution meets one of the requirements of society, namely, to make the fruits of the mystic's work available to ordinary members who have not the mystic's qualifications for at-one-ment with the deity.

The problem of membership of the group and how to decide whether or not a man was to call himself a Christian [1] also arose early. Characteristically, it hinged on the question of the therapeutic efficiency of the Christian and his brand of Christianity. The problem was brought to a head through the apparently successful therapeutic effects obtained by persons not qualified members of the group (Mark 9:38). In the instance quoted, the criterion proposed by Jesus seems to be the successful cure and its attribution by the therapist to Jesus. The issues involved are: membership of the group as itself being a symbol of status; status, expressed by the locution 'in Thy name' as a therapeutic agent; therapeutic result as a criterion of membership of the group. The solution was empirical but it accepted the criterion of therapeutic

---

[1] The modern Israeli state has met the same problem of deciding who is, or is not, a Jew.

efficiency. For the time being the test of membership seems to be twofold, namely, medical or therapeutic, and capacity for achieving results. This last requirement has been a problem throughout history. It might be described as a demand that the group leader should be able to forestall the future, confer adequacy on someone already supposed to be suitable, and guarantee his adequacy in future contingencies.

The Christian hierarchy soon found itself faced by the same problems that had defeated the rabbinical directorate. The same forces were involved: on the one side, the need to control the messianic idea and make it available to ordinary people through dogmatic formulation; on the other side, the messianic idea or its incarnation perpetually breaking through the barriers intended to control it and threatening to disrupt the society in which it became manifest. The Reformation was a spectacular example of this (see Knox, 1950).

I have used for descriptions 6 and 7 material familiar to all, for a configuration that is repeated in many forms and at many times. It is not limited to religious societies, or therapeutic societies, or artistic societies, or scientific societies, but is discernible in many societies. My intention is, however, not to express any opinion upon the nature of diverse groups. I am not purporting to write history but to formulate a pattern in picturesque C category terms; that is to say, to represent a configuration in terms that will give body to an idea that might otherwise seem to be a meaningless elaboration of abstractions. Naturally, I suppose that people other than psycho-analysts would profit from a recognition of the configuration and the underlying group to which one suspects that it belongs. But here I am concerned only as an analyst with the configuration as it might be discerned by other analysts. Descriptions 6 and 7 must not, therefore, be supposed to have a sociological or political application but to be by way of fables or mythological constructs (C category) which, if formulated with greater precision and sophistication, represent a pattern to which the human personality would be found to approximate. The fable, constructed in terms of the group, must be regarded as a pictorialization of man's inner world (Money-Kyrle, 1961). For those familiar with Kleinian theory my description can be seen as a dramatized, personified, socialized, and pictorialized representation of the human personality. It may clarify the procedure to contrast this pictorial view with the accepted morphology of classical analysis. The theory formulated in terms of ego, super-ego, and id differs in two respects. First, it is an F category formulation whereas the pictorialized formulation I am representing verbally is a C category formulation, primitive and based on sensuously derived terminology. Second, it is a theory of which the realization that approximates to it is to be found in psychopathology and psychomorphology. The realization approximating to the C category formulation is to be found in material that is superficial and easily accessible to the conscious. Its unconscious roots are to be discovered through psycho-analytic investigation.

The nature of the messianic idea can be only very approximately represented by the C category formulations I have been using. Jesus, Meister Eckhart, and Isaac Luria represent in different ways the problem of reconciling the messianic idea and the Establishment. The rabbinical directorate learned caution, so that when it had to adjust to the Lurianic doctrine, and to the injuries that Lurianic doctrine was alleged by its opponents to have inflicted on Judaism, it did not contribute to an explosion. Luria for his part insisted on his conservatism and related all he said to older authorities. Significantly, he left no writings and, when questioned by a disciple about his reasons for not setting out his teaching in book form, he replied: 'It is impossible because all things are interrelated. I can hardly open my mouth to speak without feeling as though the sea burst its dams and overflowed. How then shall I express what my soul has received, and how can I put it down in a book?' (Scholem,

1955, p. 254). Meister Eckhart wrote extensively, but the obscurity of his writing and perhaps the matter led to the condemnation as heretical of some twenty-eight propositions from his later writings. The main question seems to centre on his forthright statements of identity with the deity – 'we are transformed and changed into God'. The fate of Jesus himself has been crucifixion as a criminal on the one hand, and deification on the other. Both Isaac Luria and Jesus were alike in being followed by a proliferation of hagiographical biography; much of it, in the instance of Jesus, not being included in the canon. The common features are: containment of the messianic idea in the individual; containment of the messianic individual in the group; the problem for the Establishment that is concerned with the group on the one hand and the messianic idea and individual on the other. It is now necessary to return to the word.

Description 2 (cycle 2): If it were necessary to express descriptions 6 and 7 by one word, a choice could be made from terms such as 'religion' or 'Christianity' or 'God'. If none of these terms is considered suitable, an attempt could be made to find the suitable term by introspection. This attempt is a search in the mind for the term supposed to exist or it is a search in the meaning for the term; the latter is an instance of the meaning containing the word. The difficulties attendant on finding the word are described in the terms used by Poincaré, searching for a mathematical formula, or by Luria in the passage quoted above (p. 115). A better idea of the problem is obtained by substituting the term 'statement' for 'word' and including in its definition any act of expression whatever. In C category terms the problem is analogous to that of the sculptor finding his form in the block of his material, of the musician finding the formula of musical notation within the sounds he hears, of the man of action finding the actions that represent his thoughts. One of the peculiarities of this discussion lies in its being an example of the problem being discussed. It is an attempt to find a verbal

116

formulation to which psycho-analytic realizations approximate. I restate the problem thus: psycho-analysis, the thing-in-itself, existed. It remained for Freud to reveal the formulation embedded in it. Conversely, once formulated by Freud it remains for others (including Freud himself) to discover the meaning of the conjunction bound by his formulation.

It is necessary to postulate 'thinking' without supposing a thinker to be essential. I shall not at this point try to explain why. All thinking and all thoughts are true when there is no thinker. In contrast to this, for lies and falsities a thinker is absolutely necessary. In any situation where a thinker is present the thoughts when formulated are expressions of falsities and lies. The only true thought is one that has never found an individual to 'contain' it.

The messianic idea may be supposed to have a counterpart, the absolute truth, O, for which a thinker is not necessary. Falsity is the characteristic of thought within an individual, or thought within a container. It follows that all thought as it is ordinarily known, that is, as an attribute of the human being, is false, the problem associated with it being the degree and nature of the falsity. The lie is a falsity associated with 'morals'.

The messianic idea is a term representing O at the point at which its evolution and the evolution of a thinker intersect. The mystic, as seen in descriptions 6 and 7, is a thinker who claims the capacity for direct contact with O. The degree of falsity depends on whether the relationship with O is commensal, symbiotic, or parasitic. It is not often enough recognized that a patient in whom resistance is active can be reacting against what he feels to be a thought in search of a thinker. It is supposedly his own thought (classical resistance theory), but it does not have to be so.

The thought O and the thinker exist independently of each other. There is no reaction, or, as we should ordinarily say, identifying ourselves with the thinker, the truth has not been discovered though it 'exists'. In symbiosis the thought and the thinker correspond, and modify each other through the correspondence. The thought proliferates and the thinker develops. In a parasitic relationship between thought and thinker there is a correspondence but the correspondence is category 2, meaning that the formulation is known to be false but is retained as a barrier against truth which is feared as annihilating to the container or vice versa. The falsity proliferates until it becomes the lie. The barrier of the lie increases the need for the truth and vice versa.

The commensal position changes when thought and thinker approximate. In more usual terms, a critical situation arises when a 'discovery' threatens. It is commonly said that messianic hopes were more than usually active at the birth of Jesus and it is a matter for remark that more than one investigator often seems to be approaching a discovery at the time when a discovery is made. The resistance of the thinker to the unthought thought is characteristic of category 2 thinking. The crucial problem appears to be the relative strength of the messianic idea and the personality who is to 'contain' it. We must therefore reconsider the personality. To do this I shall use descriptions 6 and 7 as pictorial representations (C category) of the parts composing the totality of the individual, not the group. I am assuming that the reader keeps in mind existing theories of personality structure. It is not to be supposed that they are to be abandoned or even modified by what follows. Existing theories are F category formulations; what takes place in the consulting-room is an emotional situation which is itself the intersection of an evolving O with another evolving O. The description I am giving is, as it has been throughout this chapter, a C category formulation intended to bridge the gap between a unique event on the one hand and a generalized F category formulation on the other.

Description 3 (cycle 2): The messianic idea clothes itself in a variety of forms. Though it may take any form there appears to be difficulty for form and idea to achieve a symbiotic or commensal relationship. Therefore it is difficult to find a formulation by which I can convey my meaning to the reader, but I can point to the consulting-room or group where he may intuit it for himself. Similarly, I can direct him to observe the word 'cure' when he hears it; for 'within' this word he may be able to intuit the messianic idea. His attention should dwell on formulations in which he is described in positive terms; for 'within' these statements he may be able to intuit the 'contained' messianic idea. Whether the statement appears outwardly to be representing a summer holiday or a car or a person or a state in time, he should be able by degrees to intuit the frequent occurrence of the messianic idea and be persuaded of its reality and his ability to feel its presence.

When I say the reader might search the consulting-room or group, I am restricting the field of search to provide a 'container' wherein the search may be pursued without difficulty and relatively quickly. Yet it is doubtful whether intuition of a constant conjunction in the domain of psychic reality can be attainable quickly or easily. Therefore there can be no short cut for the psycho-analyst; he can hope that experience may enable him to intuit the messianic idea or recognize that this hope is itself a formulation containing it.

The idea that the messianic idea is contained within the analysis, or that descriptions 6 and 7 can be used as C category statements or formulations of the individual personality, implies that the personality can be represented by a ♂♀ relationship and that the personality has a ♀♂ relationship with a psycho-analysis. Such a formulation assists the psycho-analyst to intuit a personality, external to the psycho-analysis, which is present in the psycho-analysis only by 'hearsay'; the patient becomes a voice reporting that the messianic idea is abroad. A typical complexity of the ♀♂ relation, significant for its bearing on 'acting-out', relates to beta-elements lying outside the domain of thought proper but appearing to belong to it because they are represented 'in' the psycho-analysis by C3 statements made by the analysand. The psycho-analyst and his analysand appear, therefore, to be excluded from the domain of action and 'confined within' the domain of thought in such a way that they are not in a position to 'psycho-analyse' but only to substitute 'psycho-analysis' for psycho-analytic thinking, which is a prelude to interpretations – the psycho-analytic counterpart of action.

Psycho-analytic practice shows that the motives for any human activity are numerous and complex. They are derived from a background of sensuous desires; as fast as one is demonstrated it is apparent that further desires lie unknown. The aims of the psycho-analytic couple are arrived at by conjecture and are formulated, at least as far as the analysand is concerned, in terms representative of sensuous experience. Even the objects of curiosity are formulated in terms suitable to a sensuous background. In so far as desires can be stated they will be sensuous desires and sensuous aims, the overriding aim being to keep alive. Without exception these aims and desires are not relevant to psycho-analysis. Nor have they proved relevant in either Judaism or Christianity. Their place has not yet been taken by any formulations that are more satisfactory. So long as thinking is regarded as subordinate to the senses there is no difficulty. If thinking is a primary activity, the *aims* of contemplation or meditation are presumed to exist because thinking is tied to its genetic history as subordinate to muscular activity; similarly, muscular activity is presumed to have an aim in accord with the dominance of the pleasure principle.

It is possible that the vacuity produced by the subordination of sensuous aims to growth of a capacity for contemplation or meditation was filled, in the course of his teaching, by Jesus. But as his teaching was subjected to the twin pressures I have described, namely, annihilation by physical destruction on the one hand and divine honours on the other, we do not know what such a solution might have been. In practice the problem is shelved; thinking remains subordinate to the satisfaction of sensuous desires.

In consequence, psycho-analysis is saddled with an aim that, according to their various desires, is attributed to it by both analyst and analysand. Both are debarred from fulfilling their aim when the aim is pursued in the domain of action and the psycho-analysis is confined to the domain of thought in which thought is the only means of fulfilment. The 'conflict' is between action and thought, the counterpart, in descriptions 6 and 7, being the conflict expressed in St Augustine's refutation of the responsibility of Christianity for the fall of Rome. In the individual, demands for action and sensuous gratifications associated with physical survival conflict with the demand for mental 'activity'. The latter cannot justify itself in terms comprehensible to the former. The former cannot justify itself to the latter, for its apparatus of sensuous fulfilment is irrelevant to the domain of thought.

I have used the term 'conflict', in describing action and thought, as a reminder of the accepted view. The object of using ♀♂ is to differentiate the states of containment which, as with thought and action, prevent conflict by containing thought and containing action in a mutually exclusive commensal state. In this condition thought and action do not modify each other but persist commensally in the same personality. Actions that appear to be compulsive are in reality beta-elements confined to the domain of action and thus insulated against thoughts, which are confined to the domain of thought — which includes psycho-analysis. Similarly, thoughts are within the domain of thought and cannot be influenced by beta-elements confined within the domain of action. An apparent exception, not real, is provided by C3 elements in thoughts that appear to bring A category into the realm of thought but are only C category *records* of action; there is no conflict.

The domains of thought and action are so close, when the musculature used in talking is involved with beta-elements, that the distinction between them becomes confused. The same confusion arises if intolerance of frustration leads to a substitution of thought for action. The associated omnipotence of thought obstructs the proper use of the musculature, as a feeling of helplessness stimulated by ineffectual muscular action is often the genetic base of omnipotence: when one is active the other is present.

In the previous paragraphs I have given examples of ♀♂ associated with outside and inside. They have a psychological value in giving body to a formulation that might otherwise lack it, but the reader should seek further instances from his practice. According to his background a patient will describe various objects as containers, such as his mind, the unconscious, the nation; others as contained, such as his money, his ideas. The objects are many but the relationships are not.

The individual always displays some aspect of his personality that is stable and constant even though it may sometimes be very difficult to detect in the welter of evidence for instability; it may appear only in the regularity with which the patient attends his sessions. In this stability will be found the counterpart of what, in descriptions 6 and 7, I have called the Establishment. It will be maintained with great tenacity as the only force likely to contain the counterpart of the messianic idea. Reciprocally, the messianic idea is the only force likely to withstand the pressures of the counterpart of the Establishment in the individual. Fears of megalomanic identification with the messianic idea are associated with an inability to be at one with the omnipotent Father. The counterpart of the Establishment in the individual is not related to father or mother but can be related to fragments of both.

In the ♀♂ configuration decision is synonymous with selection for inclusion or exclusion. Thus the psycho-analyst has to decide whether to include himself in or exclude himself from various groups; to include or exclude given associations, ideas, experiences, and so on. The Establishment of the group has to decide to include or exclude certain individuals. The personality decides to include or exclude certain characteristics or, failing that, to include or exclude awareness of their existence. Dislike of the onus of decision, or awareness of responsibility for the decision, contributes to the formulation of selection procedures by which selection, like dogma and laws of science, is made to act as a substitute for judgement or a scapegoat for the guilt attendant on overtly acknowledged exercise of responsibility.

The configuration to which I have drawn attention can be seen to have a penumbra of associations which retain an illuminating function in the circumstances on which they are brought to bear. At times the light they shed distorts by over-emphasis of the irrelevant past and occlusion of the unknown (and therefore relevant) present and future. Once the constancy of the configuration is recognized its nature can be assessed and related to psycho-analytic theory. Reciprocally, theory can be reformulated when it requires readjustment.

The primitive formulation of ♀♂ in C category terms of breast and mouth, penis and vagina, has the simplicity of all C category formulations. Although descriptions 6 and 7 appear more complex, they too share the stamp of all C category formulations. Both appear to differ from the configurations represented by the Kleinian theory of paranoid–schizoid and depressive position interplay. I am unwilling to accept this apparent cleavage. The most satisfactory formulation that displays the underlying harmony relates to the practice of psycho-analysis.

The discussion of the configuration of container and contained has occupied a considerable space in this book. It may, therefore, seem surprising if, at this stage and in relatively few sentences, I describe what is perhaps the most important mechanism employed by the practising psycho-analyst. It requires less description and is relatively more easily grasped. It is for these reasons only that it occupies what may appear to be an insignificant place in this book. It is derived from Melanie Klein's descriptions of the paranoid–

schizoid and depressive positions, and to these the reader should refer.

Here, briefly, is my formulation of this matter as it concerns the practising analyst:

In every session the psycho-analyst should be able, if he has followed what I have said in this book, particularly with regard to memory and desire, to be aware of the aspects of the material that, however familiar they may seem to be, relate to what is unknown both to him and to the analysand. Any attempt to cling to what he knows must be resisted for the sake of achieving a state of mind analogous to the paranoid–schizoid position. For this state I have coined the term 'patience' to distinguish it from 'paranoid–schizoid position', which should be left to describe the pathological state for which Melanie Klein used it. I mean the term to retain its association with suffering and tolerance of frustration.

'Patience' should be retained without 'irritable reaching after fact and reason' until a pattern 'evolves'. This state is the analogue to what Melanie Klein has called the depressive position. For this state I use the term 'security'. This I mean to leave with its association of safety and diminished anxiety. I consider that no analyst is entitled to believe that he has done the work required to give an interpretation unless he has passed through both phases – 'patience' and 'security'. The passage from the one to the other may be very short, as in the terminal stages of analysis, or it may be long. Few, if any, psycho-analysts should believe that they are likely to escape the feelings of persecution and depression commonly associated with the pathological states known as the paranoid–schizoid and depressive positions. In short, a sense of achievement of a correct interpretation will be commonly found to be followed almost immediately by a sense of depression. I consider the experience of oscillation between 'patience' and 'security' to be an indication that valuable work is being achieved.

13 · Prelude to or Substitute for Achievement

'I had not a dispute but a disquisition with Dilke on various subjects; several things dove-tailed in my mind, and at once it struck me what quality went to form a Man of Achievement, especially in Literature, and which Shakespeare possessed so enormously – I mean Negative Capability, that is, when a man is capable of being in uncertainties, mysteries, doubts, without any irritable reaching after fact and reason' – John Keats.[1]

A number of aspects of the practice of psycho-analysis must now be discussed; I group them under the Language of Achievement. The quotation from Keats will serve as an introduction to the area to be covered. Language is loosely and widely defined to include behaviour of which it is sometimes said 'actions speak louder than words'. Set over against and in contrast with the Language of Achievement I consider the language that is a substitute for, and not a prelude to, action. Language of Achievement includes language that is both prelude to action and itself a kind of action; the meeting of psycho-analyst and analysand is itself an example of this language. This discussion is centred on the problem of bringing attention to bear on the realizations to which Freud's theories approximate.

Any session should be judged by comparison with the Keats formulation so as to guard against one commonly unobserved fault leading to analysis 'interminable'. The fault lies in the failure to observe and is intensified by the inability to appreciate the significance of observation. I have rarely failed to experience hatred of psycho-analysis and its

[1] 'Letter to George and Thomas Keats', 21 December 1817.

reciprocal, sexualization of psycho-analysis. These are part of a 'constant conjunction'. In C category terms: the human animal has not ceased to be persecuted by his mind and the thoughts usually associated with it – whatever their origin may be. Therefore I do not expect any psycho-analysis properly done to escape the odium inseparable from the mind. Refuge is sure to be sought in mindlessness, sexualization, acting-out, and degrees of stupor. The psycho-analyst's attention must not wander from areas of material characterized either by the Language of Substitution or by the Language of Achievement; he must remain sensitive to both. I do not claim that sensitivity can be achieved easily: the mental space available to the analysand and the material observed are subject to so many transformations that such a claim suggests inexperience of the practice of psycho-analysis. The experienced analysand finds dreams a useful stand-by because psycho-analysts are rightly expected to want to hear them. Current events can be transformed to expression in sado-masochistic terms or near psychopathological jargon; there is no limit to the forms of transformation. Experience leads to an extension of the area over which the Language of Achievement operates and therefore an extension of the area in which its operation can be recognized. We must now consider the extension of the concept of vertices in relation to both individuals in the psychoanalytical couple.

It will be remembered that the term 'vertex' can be understood as similar to 'point of view' except in certain special instances. There is a psychological or mental specificity analogous to the specificity associated with the relationship of sense organs to sense impressions. To allow for this specificity it is necessary to discard the term 'point of view' and replace it by a more abstract term such as 'vertex'. Language of Achievement is always related to a vertex whether that vertex has been determined (or evolved) or not. Since we shall consider both psycho-analyst and analysand we shall have to approach our problem by moving *outside* the field

126

usually thought of as belonging to psycho-analysis. The states of mind with which psycho-analysts deal comprise many that are generally the hunting-ground of other than psycho-analysts; for example, thieves, burglars, sexual perverts, murderers, blackmailers. Their mental world is matched by a world of external reality which caters for their states of mind by an established organization of international and commercial spying, police forces, religious organizations; the one group is matched by the other. A process of selection in Church or police force is carried out by examiners (in the instance of delinquents, by varieties of courts of law). It is intended to separate the good from the bad. Who or what is to exercise the power and what voice is to utter the Language of Achievement is a matter of consequence and has been accepted as such whether the field in which the struggle is carried on is the individual or agglomerations of individuals. Psycho-analysts accept their field to be the individual. The supposition that inhibitions should be decreased seems to be based on a view of the individual analogous to a view of the group in which democracy is a bad form of government but none the less the best.

The psycho-analyst and the analysand each have a vertex (or vertices) which, if it were known, would indicate the organization each regarded as best. Freud's scheme of id, ego, super-ego suggests one view of the organization of the personality, though there is nothing to suggest that the scheme represents a preference and not an observation.

The idea that is nourished by love develops from matrix to function in Language of Achievement; from which it can be transformed into achievement. But if the idea is subjected to splitting it may split again repeatedly, each split growing and having to be split again. Thus one gets not development but division and multiplication − cancerous, not qualitative, increase. There appears to be a great increase in ideation, but there is not, because all the ideas turn out, on inspection, to be the same one. The emotional matrix from which this springs is not envy and gratitude, but envy and greed. The idea is split over and over again and is felt to produce a quantity of splits – 'mental faeces'. Envy and gratitude, on the other hand, stimulate a desire for gain, but enable the individual to establish a good relation between what has been gained and that which has enabled him to gain it. The repudiation of the debt owed to his 'predatory' personality, and the need to continue repudiating it, exclude other parts of the personality from activity. The greed of the super-ego leads to the usurpation of the domain of reality (scientific facts) by the 'moral' outlook, and of 'scientific' laws by 'moral' laws.

The model for cancerous growth is not splitting of the object but splitting of the envy, each 'bit' then growing independently of every other 'bit'. Ostensibly these 'bits' appear as 'different' ideas. In fact they are a cover: ideas → impulses → ONE impulse. In this respect sessions can be regarded as repeating themselves, and the unchanging quality of the sessions should betray itself despite the multitudinous changes in disguise. Sometimes this state is described as a negative therapeutic reaction when it would be more accurately described as 'proliferation of fragmented envy'. If the envy were to assume an aspect of whole object it could be seen as envy of the personality capable of maturation and of the object stimulating maturation. The stimulating object is the breast (♀) or mouth (♂). They replace each other. The stimulating quality in turn replaces the stimulating object. A series of transformations is thus initiated, each a substitution for the previous one and each subject to splitting. Berkeley's criticism of Newton's mathematics is psychologically well based because it is NOT the mathematics of growth that is represented by the infinitesimal calculus and its use of concepts of infinitely small positive and negative increments – 'the ghosts of departed quantities'. It is psychologically more nearly true to regard Newton's formulation as *measurement* of restoration of whole objects than as measurement of growth. Is mathematics the Language of Achievement or of Restoration? What is required is not the decrease of inhibition but a decrease of the impulse to inhibit; the impulse to inhibit is fundamentally envy of the growth-stimulating objects. What is to be sought is an activity that is both the restoration of god (the Mother) and the evolution of god (the formless, infinite, ineffable, nonexistent), which can be found only in the state in which there is NO memory, desire, understanding.

REFERENCES

BION, W. R. (1961). *Experiences in groups*. London: Tavistock.
— (1962). *Learning from experience*. London: Heinemann.
— (1963). *Elements of psycho-analysis*. London: Heinemann.
— (1965). *Transformations*. London: Heinemann.
EISSLER, K. R. (1965). *Medical orthodoxy and the future of psychoanalysis*. New York: International Universities Press.
FREGE, G. (1950). *The foundations of arithmetic*. Oxford: Blackwell.
FREUD, S. (1911). Formulations on the two principles of mental functioning. *Standard Edition* 12.
KEATS, JOHN (1952). *Letters,* edited by M. B. Forman. 4th edition. London: Oxford University Press.
KNOX, R. A. (1950). *Enthusiasm*. London: Oxford University Press.
MONEY-KYRLE, R. E. (1961). *Man's picture of his world*. London: Duckworth.
SCHOLEM, G. (1955). *Major trends in Jewish mysticism*. London: Thames & Hudson.

Index

This index, like the rest of the book, is the outcome of an attempt at precision. The failure of the attempt will be clear; what may not be clear is the following dilemma: 'precision' is too often a distortion of the reality, 'imprecision' too often indistinguishable from confusion.